$\frac{2}{79}$ /1·75

The Neuromuscular System

Marion Therasa 1980.

Penguin Library of Nursing

General Editor
Michael Bowman

The Cardiovascular System
The Digestive System
The Endocrine System
The Female Reproductive System
The Neuromuscular System
The Respiratory System
The Skeletal System
The Urological System
The Special Senses

The Penguin Library of Nursing Series was created by
Penguin Education and is published by Churchill Livingstone.

R. S. Kocen

The Neuromuscular System

Churchill Livingstone

CHURCHILL LIVINGSTONE
Medical Division of Longman Group Limited

Distributed in the United States of America by
Longman Inc., 19 West 44th Street, New York,
N.Y. 10036 and by associated companies,
branches and representatives throughout
the world.

ISBN 0 443 01496 5

Printed in Great Britain

Contents

6 Contents

Editorial foreword

Nursing has undergone considerable change during the past decade. There have been many developments in medical science and technology, and nursing education must keep pace with these changes, not merely in principle, but in terms of the nurse's attitude and approach. These changes primarily stem from the move towards caring for the patient in the context of his entire personality – the concept of total patient care. This concept was originally underlined in the 1962 Experimental Syllabus of Training and has subsequently been mirrored with greater emphasis in the 1969 Syllabus.

The education of the nurse, as voiced nationally and professionally in this decade, has merited prominence; this is certainly underlined in the recent *Report of the Committee on Nursing* (Briggs). It now appears likely that the once rather mythical education of the nurse is now approaching reality and fulfilment. For too long there has been conflict between the service needs of the hospital and the education of the nurse.

These require effective marriage if student satisfaction and general job satisfaction of the officers concerned and, perhaps most important of all, good patient care are all to be achieved. It is hoped that this series of textbooks will go some way towards helping students achieve a better understanding, in a more interesting way, of what this concept of total patient care is all about.

The series consists of nine books; together, these books make up an integrated whole, although each can be used in isolation. Each book embraces developmental embryology, applied anatomy and physiology, pathology, treatment, nursing care, social aspects and rehabilitation of the patient. In addition, each book contains a comprehensive list of further reading for the nurse.

It is hoped that students will find much pleasure in reading these books.

Michael Bowman
Principal, Education Division, Hendon Group Training School
Examiner to the General Nursing Council for England and Wales

Preface

Patients with disorders of the nervous system form a large part of both the hospital and home-care workload. The great majority, suffering from the effects of cerebrovascular disease, are seen in general medical wards and clinics, rather than in more specialized neurological centres. More and more are able to remain at home with the support of domiciliary and social services. It is therefore important that nurses should have an understanding of the essential mechanisms of the pathological processes of neurological diseases. This does require some knowledge of the basic anatomy and physiology of the nervous system. This book attempts to cover the majority of these disorders. It is inevitable that some rare conditions should be included, if only to illustrate a point of pathological or anatomical importance, even if common conditions are discussed only briefly – usually at the expense of omitting details of management. This has been done deliberately. Management can only be learnt by personal observation and practice. It changes from time to time, as new knowledge and techniques evolve, and it also varies from place to place. Only essentials of it have therefore been outlined. For the same reason, no attempt has been made to describe any nursing procedures in detail. However, each chapter ends with a summary of the important nursing points and for this, as well as for his general advice, I am grateful to Michael Bowman, the General Editor of this series.

Chapter 1   The structure and function of the nervous system

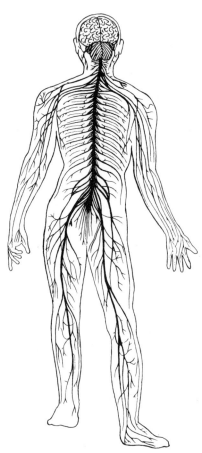

Figure 1 General picture of the peripheral nervous system

The nervous system controls the way an organism, whether animal or human, reacts to its environment. To do this, the organism must first be aware of what is going on around it. This is the function of the *sensory* part of the nervous system. The so-called *special senses* are concerned with smell, vision, hearing and taste, whilst other *sensory pathways* transmit impulses from the skin dealing with the appreciation of pain, temperature and touch, and from the joints and muscles giving information about the position of the limbs in space. Sensations are also received from internal organs such as the bowel, the bladder, the respiratory and urinary tracts, as well as from blood vessels. All movement is executed by the *motor system*. This coordinates the various striated muscles in the limbs and trunk, so that whilst some contract, others relax. The *autonomic nervous system* regulates the contraction and relaxation of smooth muscle in the walls of the blood vessels, gastrointestinal and urinary tracts and other internal organs. It is also responsible for stimulation of, and production of, secretions in the sweat, salivary and certain other glands.

Clinical neurology

Neurology is that branch of medicine which deals with disorders of the brain, spinal cord, peripheral nerves and muscles. As these disorders may involve the special senses, neurologists sometimes see patients with symptoms of disturbance of vision, balance and hearing. Neurology is closely related to other branches of medicine, as diseases of the cardiovascular system, of the endocrine organs and of metabolism may affect the function of nerve cells and produce neurological symptoms. Like the other branches of medicine, neurology is closely related to psychiatry. Psychiatric disorders may result in symptoms such as headache, impairment of concentration and of memory, and these may need to be differentiated from similar symptoms produced by neurological disorders.

At the same time, neurological symptoms due to disease of the brain or spinal cord may be aggravated, elaborated or perpetuated by anxiety or depression. For example, tremor of the hands due to a neurological disorder, whatever its precise cause, is usually aggravated by anxiety and tension, and treatment of this aspect of the patient's illness may result in considerable benefit, even if the underlying neurological cause cannot be removed. *Neurosurgery*, sometimes called *surgical neurology*, is the specialty which deals with those disorders of the nervous system amenable to surgical treatment. These include the effects of injuries, tumours and certain diseases of the cerebral blood vessels. Neurosurgeons are therefore very closely involved with the work of neurologists.

Neurological diagnosis

The purpose of making a diagnosis is firstly to allow the doctor, whenever possible, to provide appropriate treatment for the patient and, secondly, to give a prognosis, that is to indicate the eventual outcome of the disorder. This is of considerable importance both to the patient and to his family as it enables them to make plans for the future.

It is certainly not true that the majority of neurological disorders are incurable, as compared with diseases involving the other systems. There is no doubt that some crippling neurological illnesses involve the younger age groups and that, because they may not shorten life (as for instance may occur with malignant or cardiac conditions in the same age group), these patients continue to be seen in hospital for many years. Yet, in the average general medical ward, it can hardly be said that patients with chronic peptic ulcer, chronic ulcerative colitis, chronic bronchitis and emphysema, ischaemic, hypertensive and valvular heart disease, various arthritic conditions and malignant disorders are any more 'curable' than patients with disseminated sclerosis, cerebrovascular disease and some of the hereditary neurological degenerative disorders. It must be admitted, however, that neurological disabilities are often very distressing, especially when they involve the speech or the limbs or when they affect sphincter control. It is these patients, often in the prime of life, who are so often remembered because of the nursing problems involved.

The taking of the patient's history by the doctor is the most important part in the making of a diagnosis. The way symptoms begin and develop will suggest whether the illness is, for instance, due to a tumour (when the history may be that of a slowly developing and progressing disorder) or to a vascular cause (when there is usually a sudden onset and, after a time, some improvement in the symptoms). General medical history is important, as disorders of other systems may produce symptoms in the nervous system. Previous history may indicate the presence of a neurological disease with a tendency to relapses and remissions of symptoms. Many neurological diseases run in families and therefore knowledge of the family medical history is essential. Some neurological disorders may be due to exposure to toxic substances or poisons encountered at work, or perhaps to the side-effects from medicines being taken by the patient for some other condition. Finally, the doctor will attempt to make an assessment of the patient's emotional state.

The neurological examination carried out by the doctor may appear elaborate and complicated. He must assess such varying factors as the mental state, speech, function of the various cranial nerves, motor system and sensory system in the limbs. He must also examine the patient's other systems. In order to do this, it is easier to proceed in a routine fashion so that no important part of the examination is omitted. At the end of it, the doctor should have an accurate idea as to which part of the nervous system, whether the brain or spinal cord, or peripheral nerve or muscle, is the site of the disease process. He may still need, however, to carry out further investigations to make the diagnosis even more precise.

The development of the central nervous system

The brain and spinal cord lie within the bony coverings of the skull and spinal column and are known as the *central nervous system* or CNS. The sensory nerve processes which enter the CNS and the emerging motor and autonomic nerve processes together make up the *peripheral nervous system*.

The central nervous system develops from the embryonic *ectoderm*. Of the three layers of cells present in the embryo (the endoderm, mesoderm and ectoderm), the ectoderm, as well as giving rise to the skin, forms the medullary plate from which is derived the *neural tube* (Figure 2). This in turn develops into the brain structures at its forward end and the spinal cord behind. The cavity becomes the ventricular system and the central canal of the spinal cord. Alongside the neural tube lie the cells of the neural crest, which give rise to the neurones of the sensory ganglia present along the length of the spinal cord.

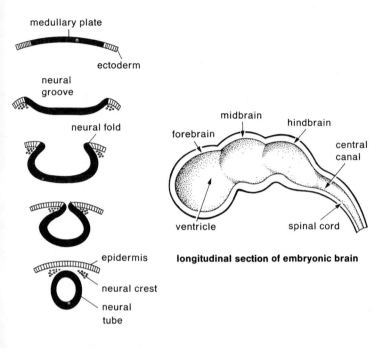

medullary plate

ectoderm

neural groove

neural fold

midbrain

forebrain

hindbrain

central canal

ventricle

spinal cord

longitudinal section of embryonic brain

epidermis

neural crest

neural tube

development of neural tube

Figure 2 The development of the central nervous system

The brain
The cerebral hemispheres

The brain consists of right and left hemispheres, each of which is subdivided into four lobes: *frontal*, *parietal*, *temporal* and *occipital* (Figure 3). Although in many ways the brain functions as a whole, there is considerable localization of function in different parts of the brain. Some of these functions can be determined by observing the effects on the patient of disease in different parts of the brain. Experiments on animals can show the effect of excising or of stimulating different parts of the brain. Thus we know that the frontal lobe is concerned with some aspects of behaviour and emotions as well as with motor function, the temporal lobe with the sensation of smell, taste and hearing, the parietal lobe with peripheral sensation and the occipital lobe with vision. It must be remembered, however, that there is considerable overlap of these different functions and that brain function is very complex. Speech is largely

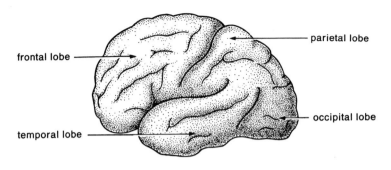

the four lobes

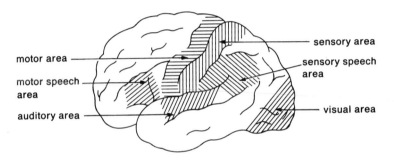

the functional areas

Figure 3 The lateral aspect of the left cerebral hemisphere

localized in the major or *dominant hemisphere*, which in right-handed people is the left one. It is less clearly localized in the right hemisphere in left-handed people. The lobes most concerned with speech are the temporal and frontal (Figure 3).

The brain-stem

Below the two cerebral hemispheres lies the *brain-stem* (Figure 4), which is the direct upward extension of the spinal cord into the skull. The upper part of it is called the *midbrain*; it is a short cylindrical structure from which the stalks of the two cerebral hemispheres arise. Within the midbrain are the nuclei of various cranial nerves, and also the *reticular formation* – one of the important coordinating areas of the CNS.

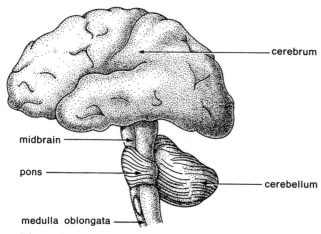

cerebrum

midbrain

pons

cerebellum

medulla oblongata

Figure 4 Parts of the brain

Below the midbrain is the *pons* (so-called from the Latin word for 'bridge'). The pons contains cranial nerve nuclei, motor fibres descending from the upper part of the brain, ascending sensory fibres and fibres connecting with the *cerebellum*. This is a rounded structure, about the size of a lemon, which is situated behind the pons, and at the same level. Its functions are largely concerned with balance and the coordination of muscular movement.

The lowest part of the brain-stem is the *medulla oblongata*. It, too, contains cranial nerve nuclei, as well as the *vital centres* (as they are called), which control activities such as heart beat and respiration.

The spinal cord

The cord begins at the *foramen magnum*, which is the largest of the apertures in the base of the skull, and runs down as far as the second lumbar vertebra. Throughout its course, it is protected by the neural arches of the vertebrae; the bony channel thus formed is called the spinal canal.

Just as twelve pairs of cranial nerves arise from the brain-stem, so thirty-one pairs of spinal nerve roots arise from the spinal cord. These emerge laterally from the cord to form spinal nerves (Figure 5) which pass through openings between the vertebrae (called the *spinal foramina*) before dividing, rejoining and then dividing again and ramifying throughout the body, as *peripheral nerves*.

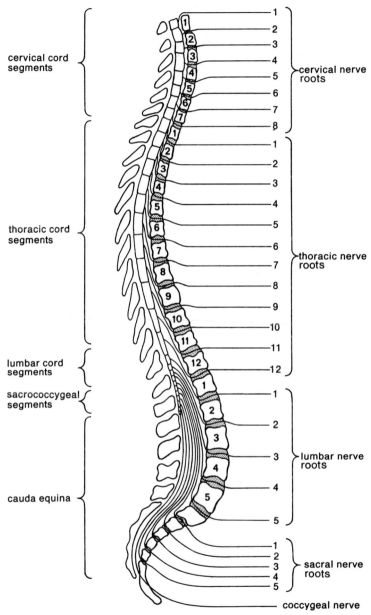

Figure 5 The spinal cord, nerve roots and vertebrae

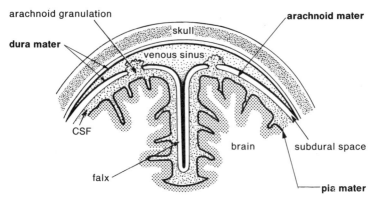

Figure 6 The three meninges covering the brain

The meninges and the CSF

The brain and the spinal cord are separated from the surrounding bone by three layers of connective tissue called the *meninges* (membranes). These are known, from the outside inwards, as the *dura mater*, the *arachnoid mater* and the *pia mater* (Figure 6). Of these, the dura mater (the outermost covering) is by far the toughest, the other two being rather flimsy. The dura mater passes down below the level of the termination of the spinal

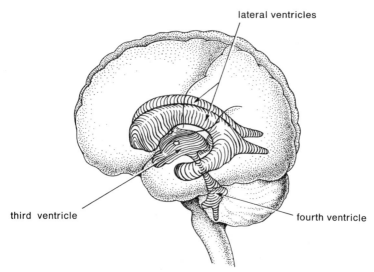

Figure 7 Lateral view of the brain, showing the position of the ventricles

cord as far as the second sacral vertebra. Between the arachnoid mater and the brain and spinal cord (that is, in the *subarachnoid space*) is the *cerebrospinal fluid* (CSF). This fluid is formed largely in spaces within the two cerebral hemispheres known as the *lateral ventricles*. The ventricular system, a series of cavities within the brain substance, (Figure 7), comprises the two lateral ventricles and the *third* and *fourth ventricles*, both of which are midline structures. The fourth ventricle lies at the level of the medulla and opens through the openings known as *foramen of Luschke* and *foramen of Magendie* into the subarachnoid space. The CSF circulates down from the ventricles, out through these foramina and over the surface of the brain and spinal cord. Eventually, it is absorbed into venous channels on the cerebral hemispheres (see Figure 6). The CSF can be tapped off from the subarachnoid space by means of the procedure known as lumbar puncture (LP).

When the brain or spinal cord are examined with the miscroscope, they are found to be composed of *neurones* (nerve cells) and *neuroglia* (supporting cells). The neurone (Figure 8) consists of a *cell body* and an *axon*, along which pass nerve impulses carrying messages to other neurones or to peripheral organs such as muscles. Axons may terminate

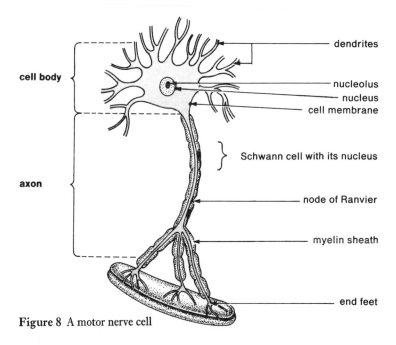

cell body

axon

dendrites

nucleolus
nucleus
cell membrane

Schwann cell with its nucleus

node of Ranvier

myelin sheath

end feet

Figure 8 A motor nerve cell

directly on other neurones or on small processes arising from them known as *dendrites*. Axons are surrounded by a white fatty substance called *myelin*.

As they pass up and down the brain, brain-stem and spinal cord, axons (together with their myelin sheaths) form the 'white matter', while the 'grey matter' is composed largely of neurones and supporting glial cells.

The motor system

The striated muscles responsible for voluntary movement receive their nerve supply from *motor neurones* which originate in the grey matter of

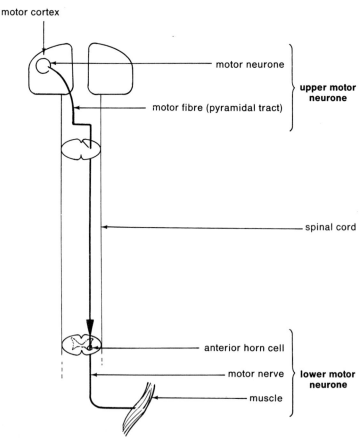

Figure 9 Motor pathways

the spinal cord or brain-stem. These *lower motor neurones*, as they are called, are under the influence of nerve fibres which originate in cell bodies lying in the motor cortex in the opposite hemisphere – these are the *upper motor neurones* (Figure 9). It is this combination of upper and lower motor neurones which is largely responsible for voluntary movement, though the lower motor neurones are also under the influence of nerve fibres originating in the cerebellum, basal ganglia and the spinal cord. The axons of the upper motor neurones which originate in the motor cortex of the cerebral hemisphere pass down in the white matter, traverse the midbrain and pons and then cross over to the opposite side. This crossing over gives the medulla a pyramidal appearance. Hence, the name *pyramidal tract* is given to these upper motor neurone fibres. Because of the crossing over, a lesion in the right cerebral hemisphere will produce left-sided weakness, and vice versa.

The lower motor neurones in the spinal cord are known as *anterior horn cells*. This name is given because grey matter in the spinal cord has the appearance of two pairs of horns (Figure 10). The anterior horn contains motor neurones whose axons leave the cord as *anterior* or *motor roots*. Each motor root combines with the posterior or sensory root to form a spinal nerve, which then emerges from the spinal canal through the intervertebral foramen.

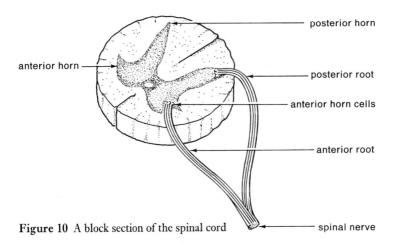

Figure 10 A block section of the spinal cord

The sensory system

The brain receives messages from the sensory nerve endings in the skin, and these bring information relating to touch, temperature and pain. Other nerve endings in joints and ligaments and in muscles convey information about joint position and movements. There is also some perception of vibration. The structure of the sensory system is quite complicated. The primary sensory neurone lies in a *ganglion* (swelling) on the posterior (dorsal) nerve root, just outside the spinal cord but within the spinal canal. It has a long axon which passes peripherally to the sensory nerve ending wherever that happens to be, whether in skin, muscle or joint. Another process passes centrally to enter the spinal cord as the sensory nerve root. Where it goes next depends on the type of sensation the nerve fibre is conveying. Fibres transmitting pain and temperature (and also

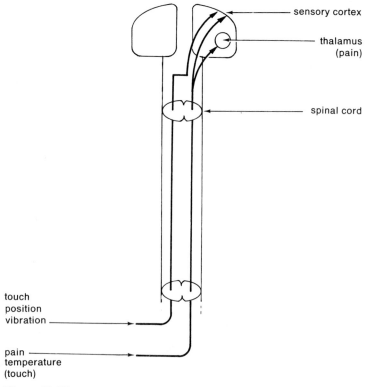

Figure 11 The mechanism for sensory perception

some of those concerned with touch) connect with other neurones whose axons then cross over to the *opposite* side of the spinal cord and pass upward towards the brain (Figure 11). There, the sensory impulses enter a structure known as the *thalamus*. Those impulses concerned with touch ascend further to the sensory cortex in the parietal lobe. On the other hand, fibres concerned with joint position and vibration sense (and some fibres conveying touch sensation) pass up the *same* side of the spinal cord in what are known as the *posterior columns*. After making connection with neurones in the lower part of the brain-stem, they cross over to the opposite side and connect with neurones in the thalamus; these carry the nerve impulses to the parietal lobe sensory cortex. Thus, eventually all the sensory fibres from one half of the body end up in the opposite thalamus and parietal lobe.

The autonomic nervous system

This part of the nervous system is outside voluntary control and acts more or less automatically. The autonomic nerves pass to involuntary or smooth muscle in the organs of the gastrointestinal tract, the bladder and the blood vessels, to glands such as the lacrimal or salivary glands and also to the pupil of the eye, controlling its size. On leaving the brain-stem and spinal cord, autonomic nerves connect with neurones which lie in ganglia, from which axons pass on to the final destination. These autonomic ganglia are situated in certain cranial nerves and in a chain by the side of the spinal column. The autonomic nervous system is further subdivided into *sympathetic* and *parasympathetic* (Figure 12). The actions of the sympathetic nervous system are largely transmitted by *adrenaline*, which is released from the nerve endings and acts on the peripheral structures. Stimulation of the sympathetic nervous system results in dilatation of the pupil of the eye, increased rate of heart beat, constriction of skin blood vessels and of rectal and bladder sphincters. Stimulation of the parasympathetic nervous system results in release of a substance known as *acetylcholine*. This produces constriction of the pupil, decreased heart rate, contraction of the intestine and bladder, and relaxation of rectal and bladder sphincters. In general the sympathetic nervous system prepares the body for action – 'fight or flight' reaction – while the function of the parasympathetic system is vegetative – in other words, concerned with the routine maintenance of bodily activities.

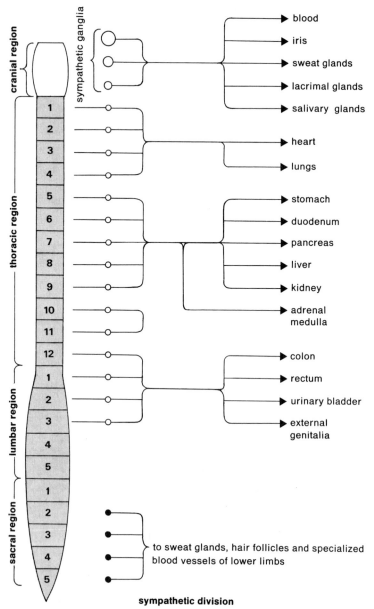

Figure 12 The autonomic nervous system

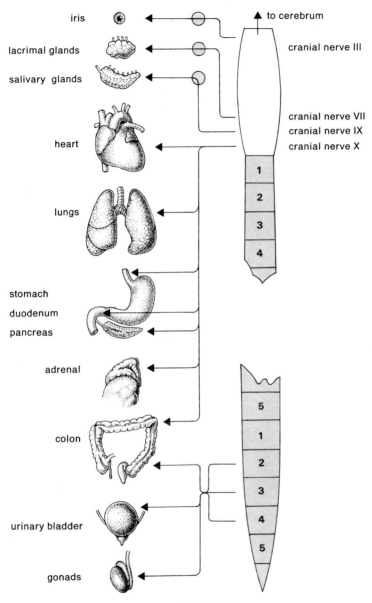

iris

lacrimal glands

salivary glands

heart

lungs

stomach

duodenum

pancreas

adrenal

colon

urinary bladder

gonads

to cerebrum

cranial nerve III

cranial nerve VII
cranial nerve IX
cranial nerve X

1

2

3

4

5

1

2

3

4

5

parasympathetic division

Summary of nursing points

The nurse should revise the anatomy and physiology of the neuromuscular system and appreciate its role in the context of the physiology of the body as a whole.

The nurse must appreciate the debilitating effects that disease of this system has on the patient. She must become skilled in detecting the signs of neurological illness and ensure that all such information is recorded and reported, so that appropriate action may be taken. In order to observe accurately and to appreciate the significance of any neurological disorders, the nurse must be fully conversant with the structure and functions of the nervous system and she must also understand the terminology used. She must accept a counselling and supportive role towards the patient in respect of the social and emotional aspects of his personality.

Chapter 2

The pathology of neurological disorders

The *pathology* of a disease means the changes seen in tissues and organs during the course of the disease. In all the disorders which may affect the body, these changes may be either *congenital* (present at birth) or *acquired*. It is usual to subdivide these changes, whether congenital or acquired:

1 *Traumatic* (i.e. due to injury). The change may be due to a physical blow, or it may be a thermal injury due to burns or excessive cold, or it may be electrical due to an electric shock.

2 *Neoplastic* (due to uncoordinated growth of cells, as in various forms of cancer). The cells involved multiply excessively and form a tumour which enlarges and destroys, by various means, the normal tissue around it.

3 *Degenerative*. These diseases may occur either because the cells die for some unknown reason, or because of failure of their blood supply to maintain their normal nutrition.

4 *Inflammatory*. The cause may be infection with microorganisms (viruses, bacteria, fungi) or larger organisms, such as parasites. It may also be due to allergy or hypersensitivity reactions.

5 *Metabolic*. In these disorders, the cells may suffer either because of the effect of some abnormal toxic substances or because of the failure of substances they require for their normal metabolism to reach them in adequate amounts. Occasionally there may be a defect in the cell due to deficiency of an enzyme or substance concerned with metabolism within the cell. This interrupts the normal metabolic pathway within the cell, leading to the accumulation of certain substances and lack of others.

The clinical manifestations of a neurological disorder, that is, the symptoms of which the patient complains and the physical signs which are found on examination, depend on two factors – the underlying *cause* of the disease and the actual *place* in the nervous system where the pathological changes are taking place. The different neurological disorders will be discussed in more detail in subsequent chapters. Here, an account will be given of some of the general changes which occur with lesions of different parts of the nervous system, including the cranial nerves.

The whole brain

The main changes which occur with disease of the cerebral hemispheres are deterioration of intellect, producing varying degrees of dementia, changes in the level of consciousness and, occasionally, emotional changes. When the left or major hemisphere is involved, there may be impairment of language function (*dysphasia*) as well as of reading and writing.

The motor system

We have already seen that this can be subdivided into the upper motor neurone system, which lies between the motor cells in the cortex and the anterior horn of grey matter in the spinal cord, and the lower motor neurone system, which consists of the neurone in the anterior horn of the cord and its axon as it emerges, first as the motor root, then as the motor fibres in the peripheral nerve. Destructive lesions of either the upper or the lower motor neurone produce interference with motor function ranging from slight weakness to complete paralysis. Whilst in both kinds of disorder there is weakness, there are four main differences which enable the doctor to differentiate between an upper and a lower motor neurone lesion.

1 In a lower motor neurone lesion there is wasting of the affected muscles.

2 In an upper motor neurone lesion the muscle *tone* (the resistance to stretching of the relaxed muscle) is increased. In a lower motor neurone lesion, the tone is normal or diminished.

3 In an upper motor neurone lesion, there is increase in the briskness of the tendon reflexes on the affected side. The tendon reflex is elicited by suddenly stretching a muscle, for instance by hitting the tendon with a reflex hammer, and observing the subsequent sudden reflex contraction of the stretched muscle.

4 On the side affected by an upper motor neurone lesion, the *plantar response* will often be 'extensor'. The plantar response (often called after Babinski who originally described it) is a movement of the big toe in response to a scratch applied to the outer border of the sole of the foot. In normal people the response is *flexor*, that is, the big toe goes down (Figure 13). In patients with an upper motor neurone lesion, the response is *extensor*, that is the big toe goes up and the little toes fan out.

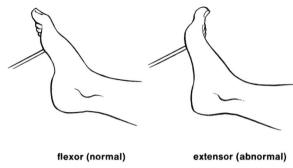

flexor (normal)   **extensor (abnormal)**

Figure 13 The plantar response

Irritative lesions may arise from the disturbance of function of neurones which are only partially damaged. When the cortical upper motor neurones are involved, involuntary movements such as localized motor convulsions may result. These will be discussed on page 92.

Both upper and lower motor neurone systems are under the influence of two other important areas in the brain. Disorders of the cerebellum produce incoordination of purposeful movements and *ataxia* (unsteadiness) of gait. Muscles controlling speech may be affected, resulting in *dysarthria* (slurring), and there may be a particular type of jerky eye movement called *nystagmus*.

The other important influence on movement comes from the basal ganglia. These consist of groups of neurones situated deep in the cerebral hemispheres. Their disorders, the most common of which is the condition known as *Parkinsonism*, will be discussed on page 107. Their main manifestations are involuntary movements, *rigidity* (increase in muscle tone) and *akinesia* (slowing down of spontaneous movements).

The sensory system

Disturbances of sensory function may also be due to destructive changes or to irritation of sensory pathways. Destructive changes produce partial or complete loss of sensations. Loss of pain sensation is known as *analgesia*.(if partial, then *hypalgesia*), and of touch as *anaesthesia* (*hypaesthesia*, if partial). Loss of position-sense from joints results in incoordination of movements (sensory *ataxia*). Irritation of sensory pathways may produce *hyperalgesia* and *hyperaesthesia* – a rather unpleasant kind of increased sensitivity to pain or touch. Feelings of tingling or pins-and-needles are known as *paraesthesiae*.

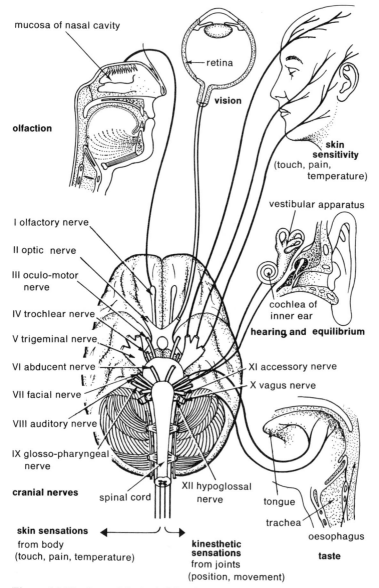

Figure 14 The base of the brain, showing the origins of the cranial nerves and the sensory routes to the brain

The cranial nerves

There are twelve pairs of cranial nerves which arise from or enter the undersurface of the brain (Figure 14). They serve very different functions and are therefore discussed individually.

The first (olfactory) nerve

The sensory nerve endings concerned with smell lie in the upper part of the nasal cavity (Figure 15). The olfactory pathway ends in the temporal lobe. The sensation of smell is responsible for the appreciation of flavours so that in conditions where it is impaired (*hyposmia*) or lost (*anosmia*), there is also impairment or loss of the ability to taste the flavour of food, except for the basic tastes of salt, sweet, acid and bitter. The most common reason for damage to the olfactory nerve is head injury. Occasionally the neurones in that part of the temporal lobe concerned with smell are partially damaged and a spontaneous sensation of smell or olfactory hallucination occurs. This is almost always an intermittent symptom lasting only for a few seconds or minutes and may be a manifestation of epilepsy arising from a lesion in the temporal lobe.

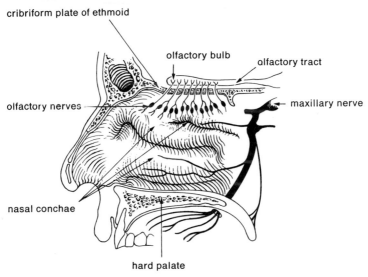

Figure 15 The olfactory nerve in the roof of the nose

The second (optic) nerve

The optic nerve connects the eye with the brain. The sensitive cells at the back of the eye, the *retina*, send processes back along the optic nerves (Figure 16) to form the *optic chiasma* and then the *optic tract* leading into the brain, where it is called the *optic radiation*. Within the brain, the fibres concerned with vision terminate in the occipital cortex, which is therefore known as the *visual cortex*. The arrangement of the optic nerve fibres results in vision to the left side of the mid-line being represented in the right occipital cortex and that from the right side in the left occipital cortex. Damage to these visual pathways at different sites along their course will result in quite different varieties of visual loss (see Figure 33).

With an ophthalmoscope, it is possible to see the back of the eye. The arteries and veins of the retina are the only blood vessels in the body which can be examined so directly, and this is of considerable importance, as their appearance often reflects the state of blood vessels in other parts

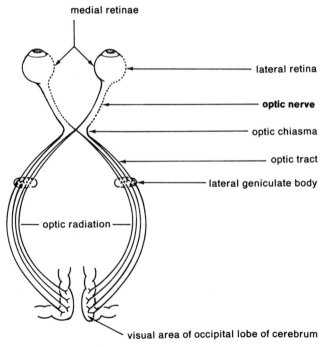

medial retinae

lateral retina

optic nerve

optic chiasma

optic tract

lateral geniculate body

optic radiation

visual area of occipital lobe of cerebrum

Figure 16 The visual pathways

of the body in conditions where blood-vessel damage may occur (e.g. hypertension or diabetes). The *optic disc* (the place where the optic nerve enters the back of the retina) can also be clearly seen with an ophthalmoscope. In conditions where intracranial pressure is raised, for instance due to an expanding brain tumour or abscess, the optic disc is swollen, a condition known as *papilloedema*. This is a very important neurological sign, as raised intracranial pressure is a potentially fatal condition requiring immediate investigation and treatment.

The ability of the eye to see (the *visual acuity*) may be recorded in a conventional way using the Snellen chart (Figure 17). The patient is asked

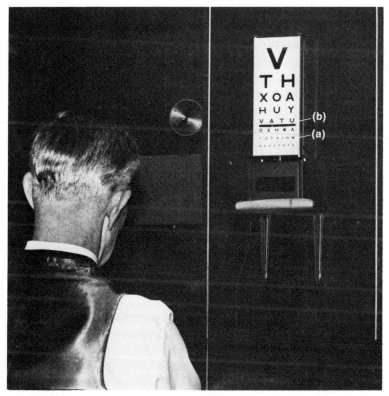

Figure 17 Testing visual acuity using the Snellen chart.
Ability to read line (a) at 6 metres represents normal vision (acuity = 6/6), whilst ability to read line (b) is equivalent to being able to read a car number plate at 25 yards (acuity = 6/12)

to read this at a distance of 6 metres, using each eye separately. The Snellen chart consists of rows of letters of decreasing size, reading down the chart. From testing large numbers of normal people, it has been established what size letter the average person can read from a variety of distances. These distances are marked below each row of letters on the chart. Thus the top letter can be read by most people at 60 metres, the one below it at 36 metres and so on. From 6 metres, the average person should be able to read the line numbered 6, and if so, his visual acuity is recorded as 6/6. If from that distance he can read only the top line, the visual acuity in that eye is recorded as 6/60, indicating that at 6 metres the person can read only what he should be able to read at 60 metres.

The third (oculomotor), fourth (trochlear) and sixth (abducent) nerves

These nerves control the *ocular muscles*, which are responsible for eye movements. The third nerve supplies four of the six external ocular muscles, the fourth and sixth nerves serve one each. The third nerve also supplies the muscle of the upper eyelid and a third-nerve palsy results in ptosis. Weakness of any of the external ocular muscles caused by a third, fourth or sixth nerve lesion results in diplopia. The size of the pupils is determined by impulses travelling in the autonomic fibres in the third nerve, the sympathetic fibres being responsible for dilatation and the parasympathetic fibres for constriction.

The fifth (trigeminal) nerve

This nerve is concerned with facial sensation and is divided into three branches, *ophthalmic*, *maxillary* and *mandibular* (Figure 18). It may be affected by a condition known as *trigeminal neuralgia* (*tic douloureux*) in which the patient complains of recurrent attacks of shooting electric-shock-like pain in the distribution of one or more of the three divisions of the nerve. The pain is brought on by touching the face, for instance when washing or even by a draught, by talking and by chewing. Its cause is unknown and, if it fails to respond to medical treatment, the involved branch of the nerve has to be destroyed by injecting it with alcohol or even by sectioning it surgically. Like other sensory nerves, the trigeminal nerve may be affected by shingles (*Herpes zoster*) which is caused by a virus. The affected area of the face becomes covered by a rash and this is often accompanied, and occasionally followed, by pain known as *post-herpetic neuralgia*. This may be very persistent and severe and results in profound depression and irritability, which aggravates it further. In cases where the

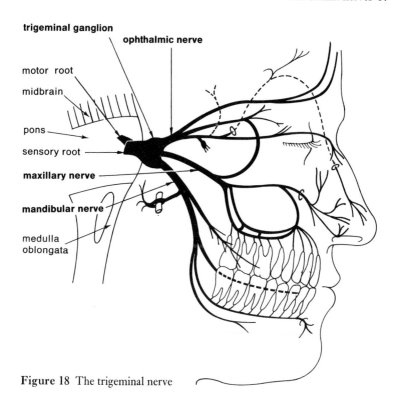

Figure 18 The trigeminal nerve

ophthalmic division of the nerve is involved, there may be impaired sensation or even complete anaesthesia of the cornea. This is a potentially very serious condition. Normally, even the smallest foreign body settling on the cornea produces pain in the eye followed by excessive production of tears, which usually results in washing it away. If this mechanism fails, then the foreign body has to be removed physically. If the cornea is anaesthetic, then the person is not even aware of the presence of any foreign body and the cornea is likely to become ulcerated. Serious infection may develop, followed by scarring and even loss of vision. An anaesthetic cornea should be protected by an eye shield or by spectacles with side protection but *not* by an eye pad applied directly to the eye which will, in itself, cause irritation of the conjunctiva of which the patient will not be aware.

The seventh (facial) nerve.

The seventh nerve supplies the facial musculature. Its nucleus lies in the pons. The upper motor neurone fibres which originate in the cerebral cortex and pass down to connect with the lower motor neurones lie, as usual, in the opposite cerebral hemisphere. However, it has been found that the motor neurones of those nerve fibres supplying the upper facial muscles receive some fibres from the cerebral cortex of their own side. This accounts for the finding that, in cases of stroke with an upper motor neurone weakness of one side of the face, the upper facial muscles are much less involved than those of the lower face, and may sometimes appear spared. The patient is therefore able to frown, wrinkle the forehead and close both eyes but, on attempting to smile, the normal muscles on the unaffected side pull the mouth over, away from the paralysed side.

In a condition known as *Bell's palsy*, the lesion in the facial nerve lies in the lower motor neurone fibres where they pass through the skull bones to the outside, and the paralysis involves both upper and lower facial muscles resulting in inability to shut the eye and even to blink on the affected side. The cause of Bell's palsy is unknown and it is fortunate that the majority of patients recover spontaneously, as there is no specific treatment. It is thought that ACTH injections or cortisone tablets given at the very beginning of the illness may improve the chance of cure. During the stage of recovery, passive exercises of the facial muscles are of value as they prevent the muscle from developing contractures. They can be performed by the patient himself, who should be shown how to pull the paralysed corner of the mouth outwards and to massage the cheek and forehead upwards. In Bell's palsy, it is important to protect the eye from foreign bodies, although, as the corneal sensation is not affected, the danger is less than with lesions of the fifth nerve. Patients should be advised to wear glasses when outdoors, even plain glass lenses if necessary. Eye infection should be treated immediately with appropriate antibiotics.

The eighth (auditory) nerve

The eighth nerve is a sensory nerve, one part of which, the *cochlear division*, is concerned with hearing and the other, the *vestibular division*, with balance. The cochlear nerve transmits information from the inner ear to the brain-stem, from where it passes upwards on both sides to the auditory cortex in the temporal lobes. A lesion of one auditory nerve will result in impairment of hearing on the affected side. The vestibular part of the nerve connects the specialized sensory endings in the inner ear with the brain-stem, where a very complicated system receives messages from the eyes, the neck muscles and the limbs and transmits them to the cerebellum and the cerebral cortex.

Disturbance of balance is a very common neurological symptom and much patience may be necessary on the part of the doctor attempting to unravel the patient's usual complaint of 'dizziness'. In lesions of the vestibular nerve and its connection in the brain, *vertigo* (see p. 99) may occur. This word describes a sensation of movement, usually of rotation of the environment around the patient (or of the patient himself). In *Ménière's disease*, which involves both the cochlear and vestibular nerve endings, there is a triad of symptoms of progressive deafness, *tinnitus* (buzzing in the ear) on the affected side, and attacks of vertigo which, when severe, may completely prostrate the patient. They may be accompanied by vomiting. The cause of this condition is unknown. In mild cases, the disturbance of balance may be diminished by tranquillizers but, in severe cases where there is already marked deafness, a destructive operation on the inner ear may be necessary to abolish the vertigo. Disturbance of balance, usually related to sudden change of posture or occurring only in certain positions of the head, known as *positional* or *postural vertigo*, may occur after certain viral infections or after a head injury. It is often difficult to separate these symptoms from those of anxiety, which frequently accompanies it.

The ninth (glossopharyngeal) nerve and the tenth (vagus) nerve

These nerves carry sensation from the back of the pharynx and upper gastrointestinal tract to the brain. The ninth nerve is concerned with transmitting taste sensation from the back of the tongue, whilst that from the anterior two-thirds of the tongue is carried in nerve fibres which join the facial nerve. Taste sensation is probably limited to the appreciation of basic tastes such as sweet, sour, salty and bitter, whilst, to appreciate the flavours, the sensation of smell is vital. The major part of the vagus nerve (Figure 19) is concerned with supplying the heart, lungs and upper gastrointestinal tract with autonomic nerve fibres and the larynx with nerve fibres to the laryngeal muscles concerned with speech.

The eleventh (accessory) nerve

This is a motor nerve supplying certain muscles in the neck. Its function can be tested by asking the patient to shrug his shoulders against resistance.

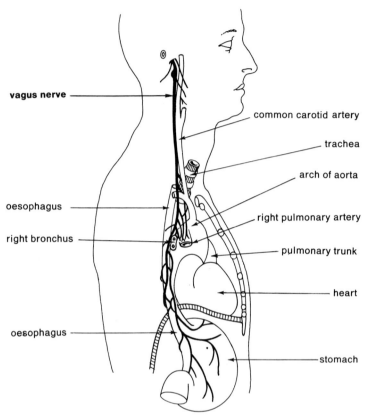

Figure 19 The distribution of the vagus nerve

The twelfth (hypoglossal) nerve

This nerve supplies the muscles of the tongue. Its function can be tested by simply asking the patient to put his tongue out straight.

Investigation of neurological patients

This has two main aims. The first is to localize the site where the disease process is occurring and the second is to try to establish what the disease process is, i.e. the *pathology* of the disorder.

In order to localize the lesion, it may be necessary to take X-rays of the skull or spine. By injecting an opaque dye into the arteries or spinal theca or air into the spaces in and around the brain to obtain contrast on the X-ray plate, a picture can be obtained showing whether these various structures are in their normal position.

In order to diagnose the cause of the disease, blood, urine and CSF, laboratory studies may be necessary. These various investigations will be discussed in more detail later on in the book.

Summary of nursing points

The nurse should appreciate the common forms of neurological disorder, together with their clinical manifestations, investigation and treatment. She should also acquaint herself with affections of the sensations of sight, hearing, smell, taste and touch. She must be fully conversant with the anatomy and physiology of the nervous system. In addition, she must be capable of making accurate observations on the patient, thereby noting any unusual features, which she must report promptly.

The observations should include those that relate to general alertness, drowsiness, affections of speech, general weakness, paralysis, incontinence and alterations in behaviour. The nurse should be aware of certain tests and examinations, such as the test for visual acuity using the Snellen chart, and also examination of the eye, using an ophthalmoscope. In patients with an anaesthetic cornea, correct care of the patient is vital to prevent irreparable damage to the eye. *A shield, and not a pad, must be used to protect the eye.*

The nurse must ensure, at all times, that the patient is reassured and anxiety lessened.

Chapter 3

Cerebrovascular disorders

The brain and spinal cord, like all other organs and tissues in the body, depend on their blood supply for nutrition and the removal of metabolic waste products. If the brain cells are deprived of blood for more than a few minutes, they die or infarct and this process is irreversible.

The cerebral circulation

The brain is supplied with blood (Figure 20) by two *internal carotid arterie.* anteriorly and two *vertebral arteries* posteriorly. These four vessels arise directly from the aortic arch or its main branches. Inside the skull, each

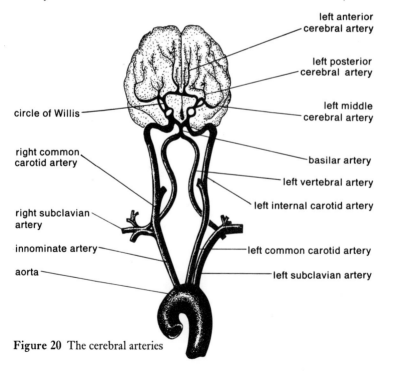

left anterior
cerebral artery

left posterior
cerebral artery

left middle
cerebral artery

circle of Willis

basilar artery

right common
carotid artery

left vertebral artery

left internal carotid artery

right subclavian
artery

innominate artery

left common carotid artery

aorta

left subclavian artery

Figure 20 The cerebral arteries

internal carotid artery divides into an *anterior* and a *middle cerebral artery*. On entering the skull, the two vertebral arteries join to form the single *basilar artery* which lies in front of the brain-stem. The basilar artery travels up and then divides into two *posterior cerebral arteries*. At the junction of the brain-stem and the base of the brain, the anterior and posterior communicating arteries anastomose (i.e. join) the anterior, middle and posterior cerebral arteries to form the *circle of Willis* (Figure 21). As long as these small joining or communicating arteries are patent (open), blockage of one or two, or even three, of the more major vessels below the level of the circle of Willis will not deprive the two hemispheres of their blood supply. However, obstruction of one of the major vessels above the circle of Willis is likely to result in infarction or death of the brain tissue supplied by that artery. This is because there is very little, if any, anastomosis of the terminal branches of the intracerebral arteries.

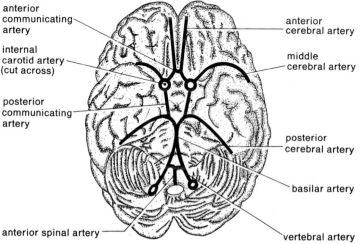

Figure 21 Basal view of the brain, showing the circle of Willis

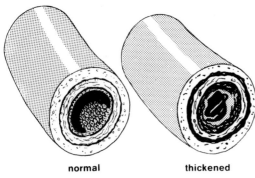

normal   **thickened**

Figure 22 Thickening of the artery walls

After travelling through brain capillaries, the blood enters a system of veins which join to form venous sinuses. These ultimately return the blood through the jugular veins to the heart.

Pathology of cerebrovascular disorders

Degenerative pathological changes take place in blood vessels throughout the body at an increasing rate with age. In arteries, the main effects of these changes are twofold. The first is a thickening of their walls (Figure 22) leading to narrowing and a reduction in the amount of blood going

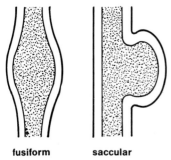

fusiform   **saccular**

Figure 23 Types of aneurysm

through them, and the second is weakening of their walls which may result in either an *aneurysm* (a localized expansion) (Figure 23) or a rupture. These processes of thickening, narrowing and weakening occur simultaneously and certain diseases such as *hypertension* (high blood pressure) and *diabetes mellitus* accelerate them. Diet may also play a part in their development. These changes are known as *atheroma*.

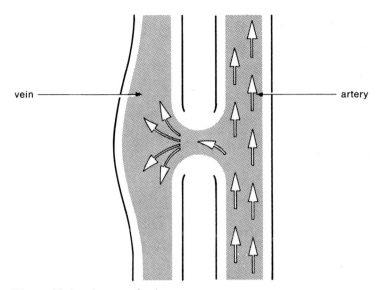

Figure 24 Arteriovenous fistula.
The arrows indicate the path taken by the blood in passing directly from the artery to the vein

Apart from such degenerative changes, blood vessels may be affected by congenital disorders which result in various abnormalities. These may be congenital weakening of arterial walls resulting in congenital aneurysm formation, or congenital communications between arteries and veins leading to the formation of an *arteriovenous fistula* (Figure 24). Arteries may also be involved in inflammation (*arteritis*) and this can also lead to their thickening and obstruction and rupture. Trauma in the form of head injury is also an important cause of rupture of intracranial vessels, particularly those lying in relation to the covering membrane of the brain, the dura mater, either just outside (*extradural*) or just inside (*subdural*). Extradural and subdural haemorrhage will be considered in more detail in Chapter 5.

Intracranial aneurysm and subarachnoid haemorrhage

We have already mentioned that the wall of an artery may occasionally be weakened and an aneurysm (swelling) may form on it. This may occur because of a congenital weakness, or it may be secondary to atheroma. It usually occurs in the section of the artery after it has pierced the meninges but before it has entered the brain, in the so-called subarachnoid space. This space lies between the arachnoid membrane, the innermost of the meninges and the surface of the brain and spinal cord (see Figure 6).

Most commonly, aneurysms arise in one of the arteries forming the circle of Willis. They may expand and compress the structures lying close to them. Expanding aneurysms in the circle of Willis usually press on one or several of the cranial nerves in their vicinity. Pressure on the third cranial nerve will result in *ptosis* (drooping of the eyelid), paralysis of some of the ocular movements causing *diplopia* (double vision) and *mydriasis* (dilatation of the pupil). Pressure on the fifth nerve may produce either pain or numbness in the face. Pressure on the second nerve or on the optic chiasma will produce visual failure and even blindness.

Rupture of an intracranial aneurysm results in a *subarachnoid haemorrhage* (Figure 25). This usually begins suddenly with severe headache, vomiting, *photophobia* (dislike of bright lights), and sometimes loss of consciousness. The main physical sign is neck stiffness, that is, resistance to flexion. This is thought to arise from irritation of the nerve endings in the meninges by the free blood present in the subarachnoid space, where previously only cerebrospinal fluid flowed. The diagnosis of a subarachnoid haemorrhage is confirmed by examining the cerebrospinal fluid, obtained by a lumbar puncture (see p. 74). Instead of the normal

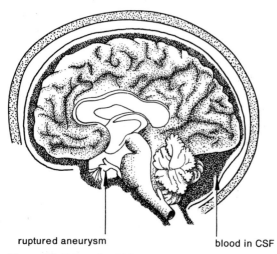

ruptured aneurysm   blood in CSF

Figure 25 Subarachnoid haemorrhage

clear colour, it is uniformly blood stained and, when allowed to stand for the red cells to settle to the bottom of the bottle, it is *xanthochromic* (yellowish) indicating that the blood has been present for at least some hours. This differentiates it from a blood-stained cerebrospinal fluid obtained by a traumatic tap because the lumbar puncture needle has entered a small blood vessel.

Once a subarachnoid haemorrhage has occurred, there is no specific treatment except bed rest for a period of three to four weeks to allow the ruptured vessel to heal. However, about one-third of patients die in this condition and another one-third run the risk of recurrence and possibly death. In those who survive, there may also be permanent neurological damage because some degree of destruction of brain tissue may occur

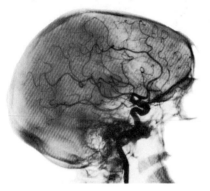

lateral view, arterial phase

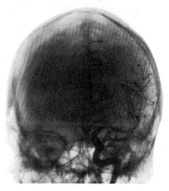

antero-posterior view, arterial phase

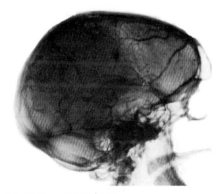

lateral view, venous phase

Figure 26 Normal carotid arteriogram

during the haemorrhage. It is because of this high possibility of recurrence and risk of death or permanent disability that investigations are usually carried out to determine the site of the rupture before deciding whether some form of treatment may prevent such a recurrence.

The cerebral arteries are outlined (Figure 26) in the investigation known as an *arteriogram*. A radio-opaque dye, injected into either the carotid or vertebral artery in the neck, travels into the intracranial part of the vessels and will demonstrate the presence of an aneurysm (Figure 27).

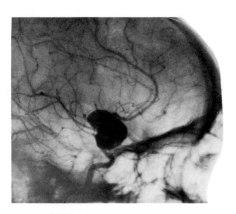

lateral view

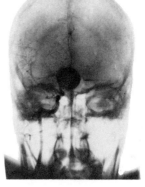

antero-posterior
view

Figure 27 X-rays showing an aneurysm

There is a variety of surgical procedures which are thought to reduce the possibility of recurrence of a subarachnoid haemorrhage. Which operation is carried out depends on such general factors as the patient's age and general condition, level of blood pressure and state of blood vessels elsewhere, and the exact site and size of the ruptured aneurysm. Some aneurysms may have a metal clip placed across their necks. Others may be wrapped around with muscle or connective tissue taken from the leg, or with plastic material. Sometimes the carotid artery in the neck may be tied off to reduce the pressure within the aneurysm above. This procedure does not usually result in an infarction of a cerebral hemisphere as the anastomosing arteries in the circle of Willis will normally take over the blood supply. As both the procedure of arteriography, and especially the surgery which may follow, carry some risk to the patient, many factors must be considered by the neurologist and neurosurgeon before they are undertaken.

Strokes

The term *stroke* means the development of weakness or sensory loss or impairment of speech or of brain–stem function as a result of a sudden disturbance of blood supply to a part of the brain. This clinical picture is the result of blockage or rupture of an intracranial blood vessel. There are three basic ways in which this may occur: *embolism* and *thrombosis* (both of which produce infarction of brain tissue) and *haemorrhage* (Figure 28).

Cerebral embolism means the sudden obstruction of a blood vessel by a small blood clot or embolus which originated elsewhere and travelled up an artery until its size was too large to enable it to pass on any further. An embolus may form in the heart or on the wall of a large blood vessel such as the aorta or carotid artery in the neck, on scarred or fibrous tissue or in areas affected by atheroma. In the heart, it may arise where there has been damage to the heart wall or valves from such conditions as rheumatic heart disease or following myocardial infarction. When an embolus blocks an artery there is usually death of the brain cells (infarction) in the area which it supplies with blood. At the edges of the infarct, some recovery of partially destroyed brain tissue may ultimately take place. Occasionally, emboli may be so fragile that they rapidly break up almost as soon as they have blocked a small artery and before any permanent damage to the

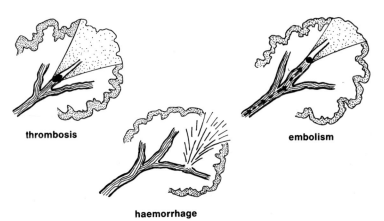

thrombosis

embolism

haemorrhage

Figure 28 Types of cerebrovascular accident and their effect upon the brain

tissues has occurred. This gives rise to so-called transient *ischaemic* attacks (*ischaemia* means reduction of blood supply). This will show itself as attacks of weakness, sensory disturbance or double vision, or other neurological symptoms due to a disturbance of cerebral circulation lasting for several minutes or perhaps even a few hours with eventual complete recovery of function. Occasionally the ophthalmic artery (a branch of the internal carotid), is the site of recurrent emboli, resulting in repeated episodes of transient blindness in one eye.

Cerebral thrombosis describes the formation of a blood clot or thrombus within the lumen of a cerebral artery. This may happen if the process of atheroma becomes so severe that the thickening of the arterial wall eventually leads to such slowing of the blood flowing through it that it eventually clots. Just as in the case of an embolus, there is infarction of brain tissue beyond the obstruction. A common site for occlusion of an artery by a thrombus is in the internal carotid artery near its origin from the common carotid artery in the neck. We have already seen that in people with healthy patent arteries, the circle of Willis is able to take over the blood supply of all the smaller arteries which arise about its level. However, in people with atheromatous arteries, the communicating vessels in the circle of Willis may be so narrow (or even completely occluded) that, should thrombosis occur in the internal carotid artery, part of the brain which it supplies with blood may infarct.

A *cerebral haemorrhage* is due to the rupture of an artery within the brain substance. This happens when the arterial wall is weakened – almost always due to a persistently raised blood pressure (hypertension).

The clinical manifestation of these three forms of stroke may differ slightly. Cerebral thrombosis tends to develop more slowly than either cerebral embolus or haemorrhage. It may take several hours to reach its maximum effect, whereas the other two develop within minutes. Cerebral haemorrhage is most likely to be associated with loss of consciousness. It is also the type of stroke most likely to result in death, either immediately or within a few hours of onset. Following an infarction due to either cerebral thrombosis or cerebral embolus, some recovery of function usually takes place. This is due to some extent to the fact that around an infarct there is a greater or smaller zone of only partially damaged neurones and nerve fibres and of cerebral oedema. This is caused by outpouring of plasma from partially damaged capillaries in the infarcted area and causes further damage to the neurones at the edge of the infarct. These partially damaged neurones, which may ultimately recover, account for some of the clinical recovery seen in patients with strokes. Some of the recovery is also due to the remaining healthy neurones taking over the function of those which have died, but this probably accounts for only a small part of the improvement seen.

Treatment

An unconscious patient should be nursed in the usual way: whatever the cause of the unconsciousness, it is most important to maintain a clear airway. The mouth must not be obstructed, the tongue should not fall back to block the upper part of the throat (Figure 29), and secretions from the nose, mouth, larynx and trachea should not be allowed to enter the lungs. To maintain a clear airway, the patient should be nursed in the half-prone position. He should be half on his front, half on his side, with his head turned to one side to keep the nose and mouth clear, and with his trunk sloping down towards the head, so that fluid will drain out of the trachea instead of into the lungs. The trunk may be propped in position by pillows, or the foot of the bed may be slightly raised by blocks. Chest physiotherapy is vital at this stage to prevent the development of pneumonia.

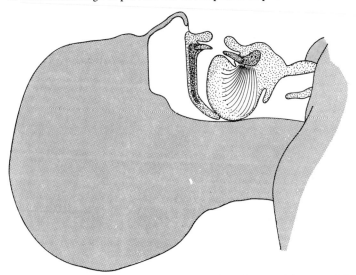

Figure 29 The airway of an unconscious patient obstructed because of the loss of tone in his jaw and flexion of his neck

Nutrition of an unconscious patient is maintained through a nasogastric tube or intravenously (but it is difficult to give sufficient calories this way). The bladder is drained by a catheter, although drainage may be accomplished by an external apparatus attached to the penis. Early mobilization of patients will prevent the stiffening of paralysed muscles. Physiotherapy is an essential part of rehabilitation to relieve muscle spasticity, prevent the development of contractures and enable the patient to achieve maximum use even in paralysed and spastic limbs. Speech therapy may help some patients with *dysphasia* and *dysarthria*. The mental aspect must never be forgotten. Depression is a common result of a stroke and will obviously prevent full recovery. In rehabilitating patients and attempting to reorganize their life at home, much help may be obtained from occupational therapists and the social services.

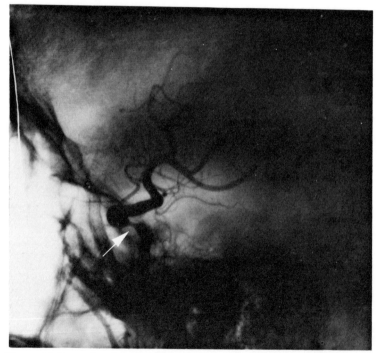

Figure 30 X-ray showing carotid stenosis (arrowed)

Unfortunately, specific medical treatment has, on the whole, little to offer the majority of patients with a stroke, whatever its mechanism. Where an embolus from the heart has occurred, anticoagulant drugs which reduce the tendency to intravascular clotting may diminish the possibility of further emboli. They have also been used in treating patients with transient ischaemic attacks, but it is difficult to assess their effect. Cerebral thrombosis is not amenable to any active treatment, but it is important to investigate such patients to exclude predisposing conditions such as hypertension, diabetes and disturbances of blood lipids and cholesterol. The same applies to those who recover from a cerebral haemorrhage. Occasionally surgical evacuation of the blood clot may relieve the symptoms in patients with intracerebral haematoma.

If a patient is suspected of having *stenosis* (narrowing) of the internal carotid artery in the neck, this may be demonstrated by carotid arteriography (Figure 30). The stenosed segment can be replaced surgically by an arterial or synthetic graft.

Arteritis

Inflammation of the arterial wall or sometimes even of structures around it may result in thrombosis by causing thickening of the walls and narrowing of the arterial opening inside them. Probably the most common cause of arteritis causing cerebral thrombosis and infarction is syphilis. This will be discussed on page 79.

Another important condition is *temporal arteritis*, so called because it characteristically involves the temporal arteries in the scalp. It is also known as *giant cell arteritis* because, under the microscope, the cells in the inflammatory tissue in the arterial walls are very large and have more than one nucleus. Temporal arteritis may involve the arteries supplying the eye and, if these are occluded blindness results. The disease typically occurs in people aged over sixty and the main symptoms are headache, pain and extreme tenderness over the arteries in the scalp. The *erythrocyte* (red blood cell) *sedimentation rate* (ESR) is very high and the diagnosis is established by taking out a small portion of temporal artery under local anaesthetic and finding the typical changes under the microscope. Treatment consists of the administration of corticosteroids for as long as there is headache and the ESR is raised. The disease usually settles within a variable period of time.

Summary of nursing points

The cerebral circulation is a vital one; should the blood supply to any part of the brain be cut off, the resulting effects will be serious and may include loss of consciousness, permanent cerebral damage and, in the extreme, death. These conditions may occur without prior warning, and with accompanying dramatic effects. Common cerebrovascular conditions include aneurysm, haemorrhage, embolism and thrombosis.

The nurse must appreciate the importance of these conditions, together with their clinical manifestations and treatment. The clinical manifestations will depend on the site and severity of the lesion. The nurse must be conversant with the nursing care of the unconscious patient; this will include the position of the patient (usually semiprone) and the maintenance of a clear airway. The patient's position must be changed regularly – usually every two hours. His toilet must be performed regularly and every effort made to prevent pressure sores.

The following observations must be made and recorded: temperature, pulse, respiration and blood pressure, fluid balance, excretions, degree of paralysis and changes in behaviour.

The nurse may have to prepare the patient for surgery, should this be indicated. It is vital that she understands the post-operative regime, in an effort to prevent complications and ensure the patient's comfort.

Chapter 4

Tumours of the nervous system

The growth of tumours

The great majority of cells which make up the various organs and tissues of the body are in a constant state of growth, development, multiplication and finally death. The life-span of a cell varies. A red blood corpuscle survives for about one hundred and twenty days, whereas some cells in the skin and gastrointestinal tract may survive for only a few hours before dying and being replaced by others. As far as is known, the neurones in the brain and spinal cord do not proliferate after birth. When the mechanism controlling the rate of multiplication of a group of a particular kind of cells breaks down, they may proliferate in an uncontrolled way giving rise to a tumour or a *neoplasm* (new growth). This is an abnormal mass of tissue whose rate of growth is uncontrolled and exceeds that of the normal cells of that type.

In any organ, the tumour which originates from cells normally present in that organ is known as a *primary tumour*. When a tumour grows, it expands and extends into the rest of the organ and may even spread into neighbouring organs. Those tumours which are surrounded by a connective-tissue capsule and remain confined to the organ in which they have arisen are known as *benign tumours*. The tumours which *metastasize* (spread) into neighbouring organs either directly or through blood vessels or lymphatics are known as *malignant tumours*. If a tumour spreads to other organs it is then said to have given rise to *secondary tumours* or metastases. Benign, encapsulated tumours can usually be removed at operation. Malignant tumours which do not have a capsule are usually never completely removable, even from their organ of origin.

In the nervous system, tumours may occur in the brain, the spinal cord and the peripheral nerves. Primary tumours usually arise from the various kinds of supporting cells such as astrocytes or cells in the meninges. Tumours arising from the neurones themselves are very rarely seen, and then usually in children. Secondary tumours may often affect the brain or the spinal cord. The primary site is usually the bronchus, breast or gastrointestinal tract. It is not uncommon for a patient to go to the doctor with symptoms of a secondary tumour in the brain without any symptoms from the underlying primary neoplasm.

Intracranial tumours

The symptoms and signs of an intracranial tumour fall into two groups – those due to raised intracranial pressure and those due to the direct involvement of the brain and cranial nerves – the focal signs and symptoms. Expanding brain tumours give rise to raised intracranial pressure because the skull is a rigid container. The symptoms of raised intracranial pressure are headache, vomiting and drowsiness. A rapidly growing tumour is more likely to produce these symptoms than a slowly growing one, which gives the intracranial structures months or even years to adjust to its slow expansion. The headache is typically present on waking, relieved by upright posture, aggravated by straining and may be accompanied by vomiting. The chief sign is *papilloedema* (swelling of the optic discs), visible at the back of the eye with an ophthalmoscope. This may be accompanied by episodes of transient blurring of vision.

The main dangers of raised intracranial pressure are progressive impairment of consciousness and irregularity of the heart and respiratory rhythms. Raised intracranial pressure will result in pressure on the brain-stem from above, since the skull is a closed cavity. The brain-stem becomes compressed and distorted as it passes through the opening in the tentorium which separates the cerebral hemispheres above from the cerebellum in the posterior fossa below. The brain-stem may also be compressed from the side by an expanding lesion in one cerebral hemisphere which will displace the temporal lobe medially against the brain-stem. Compressions of the brain-stem will result in increasing drowsiness because of interference with the function of those neurones in the reticular formation which are concerned with consciousness. There will also be disturbance of functions of the centres in the medulla responsible for the heart rate and respiratory rate. In addition, the third cranial nerve (which passes through the tentorial opening) may also be affected and this will result in *mydriasis* (dilatation of the pupil), *ptosis* (drooping of the eyelid) and *diplopia* (double vision) because of paralysis of ocular movements.

The focal symptoms of an intracranial tumour are usually due to a combination of destructive and irritative effects. Destructive effects in the cortex of the cerebral hemispheres may cause weakness of the limbs, sensory impairment and, if on the left hemisphere, *dysphasia* (language disturbance). Focal symptoms may also be due to compression of isolated cranial nerves. Irritative effects result in various types of epilepsy, the particular features depending on where the tumour happens to be. Tumours in the cerebellum produce *ataxia* (disturbance of balance and coordination), *dysarthria* (slurred speech) and *nystagmus* (jerky eye movements).

Glioma

For reasons which are not known, nerve cells do not themselves give rise to tumours, but tumours of the supporting or glial cells are not uncommon These *gliomas*, as they are called, are the most common primary brain tumours (Figure 31). The two main types of glial cells, the astrocytes and

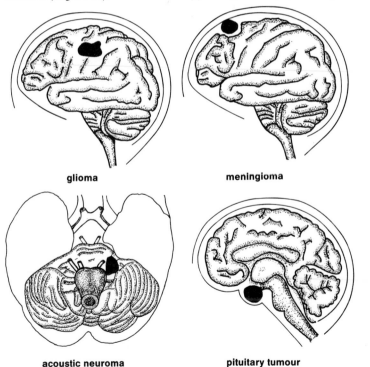

glioma

meningioma

acoustic neuroma

pituitary tumour

Figure 31 Some varieties of intracranial tumours

oligodendrocytes, give rise to *astrocytomas* and *oligodendrogliomas*, respectively. These are malignant tumours, without a capsule, which spread by infiltrating the brain tissue. They do not metastasize to other organs, but they cannot be removed completely from their site in the brain. Some may grow rapidly and cause death within a few weeks of onset of symptoms, whilst others may take years to produce significant damage. Symptoms may sometimes be relieved by partial removal, and occasionally the growth of the tumour may be slowed by radiotherapy.

Meningioma

This is the second most common primary brain tumour (Figure 32). It arises from the connective tissue cells of the meninges covering the brain.

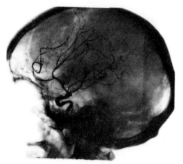
arteriogram, arterial phase

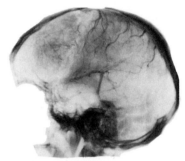
arteriogram, venous phase

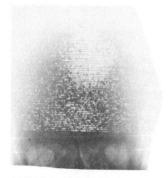
gamma scan, lateral view

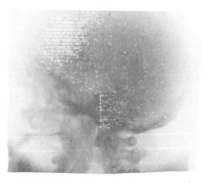
gamma scan, antero-posterior view

Figure 32 Meningioma.
The arteriograms show the blood vessels displaced by the tumour, and the gamma scans show increased uptake of radioactive isotope in the tumour area

It therefore compresses the brain from outside and, being encapsulated, does not infiltrate the brain tissue and can usually be removed completely by the neurosurgeon. Occasionally complete removal may be impossible if the tumour lies close to a vital artery or venous sinus and cannot be separated from it without the risk of unstoppable haemorrhage.

Acoustic neuroma

This benign tumour arises from the supporting or neurolemma cells of the eighth cranial (auditory) nerve. It produces deafness and, if it compresses the seventh and fifth nerves lying close to it, facial paralysis and numbness. It also compresses the cerebellum resulting in ataxia, dysarthria and nystagmus. By obstructing the outflow of the CSF from the ventricles, it eventually gives rise to raised intracranial pressure. Its complete removal may be difficult because it lies very close to the medulla and pons; during the operation, centres concerned with cardiac and respiratory control which lie in that part of the brain-stem may be damaged, resulting in cardiac or respiratory arrest.

Pituitary gland tumours

The two main effects of these are compression of the optic chiasma and disturbance of the function of the pituitary gland. Chiasmal compression produces initially *bitemporal hemianopia* (Figure 33) and eventually

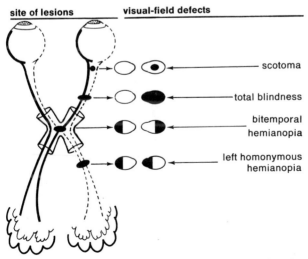

site of lesions   **visual-field defects**

scotoma

total blindness

bitemporal hemianopia

left homonymous hemianopia

Figure 33 Lesions of the visual pathways and the resulting visual-field defects

bilateral blindness. Hypopituitarism or underactivity of the pituitary may result from impaired production of the main pituitary hormones. Occasionally a particular type of pituitary tumour may give rise to excessive secretion of pituitary hormones with the resultant development of acromegaly. Another type of pituitary tumour may cause Cushing's syndrome. Pituitary tumours (Figure 34) can usually be removed either completely or partially and they are fairly sensitive to deep X-ray therapy.

Brain tumours in children

Whilst children may develop any of the tumours mentioned above, they may also develop some arising from cells which do not normally persist into adult life. One of these, a *craniopharyngioma*, arises in close relation to the pituitary gland and optic chiasma and its local effects are due to

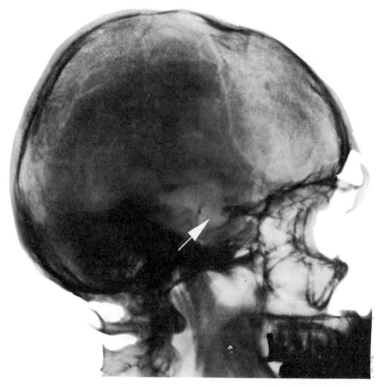

Figure 34 X-ray showing a pituitary tumour; the enlarged pituitary fossa is arrowed

compression of these structures. It may be partially removed and takes many years to recur. Another, *medulloblastoma*, arises in the cerebellum. Unfortunately, this tumour is not amenable to either surgery or to deep X-ray therapy.

Investigations
When an intracranial tumour is suspected, a skull X-ray may show evidence of raised intracranial pressure such as enlargement of the pituitary fossa, and occasionally calcification in the tumour. An electroencephalogram may show a localized abnormality over part of one hemisphere. A carotid arteriogram may localize the tumour by showing displacement of related blood vessels. An air-encephalogram (Figure 35) or ventriculogram may also localize it by demonstrating displacement

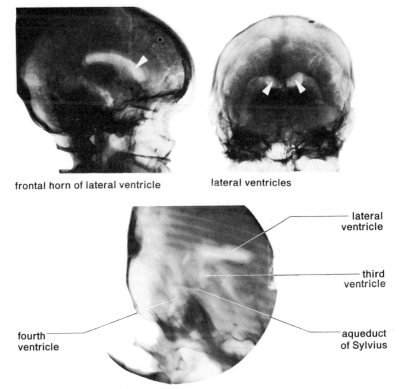

frontal horn of lateral ventricle   lateral ventricles

lateral ventricle

third ventricle

aqueduct of Sylvius

fourth ventricle

Figure 35 Air-encephalograms

of the cerebral ventricles. A radio-isotope brain scan may show an area of increased isotope uptake over the lesion.

Spinal cord tumours

These may also be primary or secondary, the latter being more common. Primary tumours may be benign or malignant and, depending on whether they are outside or inside the dura, they are called *extradural* or *intradural*. Intradural tumours may be intramedullary (within the spinal cord itself) or extramedullary.

Because the space within the spinal canal is small, the enlarging tumour soon produces compression of the spinal cord (Figure 36). This is an emergency of the greatest importance. If the spinal cord is severely compressed for more than several hours, with progressively increasing interruption of the ascending and descending pathways, then even if the compression is relieved, the already damaged fibres may not recover. The shorter and the more rapidly progressive the history, the more essential is the need for rapid investigation and relief of compression.

The chief symptoms and signs of spinal-cord compression are due to the interruption of those pathways in the spinal cord that are concerned with movement, sensation and the function of the bladder and bowel. Pressure on the pyramidal tract results in upper motor neurone weakness of the limbs below the compression, and similarly there is diminution and even complete loss of all forms of sensation below the level of the lesion.

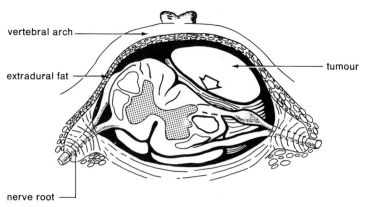

Figure 36 Spinal cord tumour

Earlier, during the irritative stage, there may be abnormal sensations (*paraesthesiae*), such as pins-and-needles. At the level of the tumour, pressure on the sensory roots may give rise to root pains in their distribution over the body or limb. The effect on the bladder and bowel is more complex. Usually, in progressive lesions there is at first increased frequency and urgency of micturition. Later, there is retention of urine and, as the bladder becomes insensitive, it enlarges and overflows, leading to chronic retention with overflow incontinence. Complete transection of the cord is immediately followed by acute retention of urine.

The longer these various symptoms are allowed to persist, the less likely is recovery to occur. Patients with suspected spinal tumour must therefore be investigated early. Plain X-rays of the spine may show erosion of bone. A myelogram, in which a radio-opaque dye is injected into the subarachnoid space through a lumbar puncture needle, may demonstrate blockage to the flow of the dye when the patient is tipped up and down on an X-ray table.

Primary benign tumours compressing the spinal cord may be either meningiomas or neurilemmomas, and these can usually be removed completely. Primary malignant tumours and secondary tumours cannot be removed completely, but even partial removal may result in some relief of symptoms whilst the patient remains alive. Unless the patient's general condition contra-indicates it, then surgery is performed to relieve spinal cord compression by removing the laminae of the vertebrae (*laminectomy*) and excising the tumour completely if possible.

Summary of nursing points

The principal primary tumours of the nervous system are glioma, meningioma, acoustic neuroma and pituitary gland tumours, whilst children may also suffer from craniopharyngioma and medulloblastoma. The nurse must be familiar with the clinical manifestations of all these tumours – headache, vomiting, drowsiness, weakness of the limbs, irregularities of the heart and respiration, and even personality changes.

Observations on the patient must include his emotional state, level of consciousness, reaction to stimuli, temperature, pulse, respiration, blood pressure, posture and balance. The nurse must be able to prepare the patient for such examinations as arteriogram, ventriculogram and encephalogram.

The patient with paraplegia must have scrupulous nursing care. Important points are the nursing position, care of the skin, general toilet and position of the limbs. Paralysed limbs should be supported in the most comfortable position. The bed should be made up with a firm mattress, and a side rail should be provided to prevent the patient falling out of bed. Passive movements of the affected limbs should be carried out as often as possible, and the nurse should give ample and regular reassurance to keep up the patient's morale. Every effort should be made to rehabilitate the patient by education and to give him constant social and emotional support.

Chapter 5   Head injuries

Head injuries and unconsciousness

With the ever-increasing use of the motor car and the rising accident rate, head injury is probably the most common cause of brain damage seen in hospital wards. The majority of victims are admitted purely for observation because of the danger that they might develop a fatal complication some hours later. It is extremely important therefore for nurses watching over such patients to appreciate this. The main indicator of brain damage is the level of consciousness, probably better called the level of responsiveness, of the patient. Whilst there is obviously a whole range of states between full consciousness and complete coma, it is unfortunately true that descriptions such as drowsiness, semicoma and stupor are not clearly defined and are best avoided as they may mean different things to different observers. This is particularly important if the patient is moved from one hospital to another.

A precise but brief description of the degree of responsiveness of the patient, that is, what he is and is not able to do, is essential. A fully conscious patient reacts in a normal rational way to spoken commands. A less conscious one appears drowsy but is readily rousable, can answer questions, and obey simple commands rationally. A patient who is rather deeper into unconsciousness does not obey commands but responds to a painful stimulus by withdrawing the part of the body to which pain is applied and also by trying to push away the pinching or pressing hand of the examiner. In an even more deeply unconscious patient, there is no purposeful response to pain but perhaps only a moan and a stiffening of the painful limb or other limbs. Finally, when the depth of coma is profound, there is no response whatever to pain except perhaps a completely involuntary reflex extension of all the limbs. Allowance must, of course, be made for the fact that the patient may be deaf or dysphasic, so that he may not be able to appreciate the meaning of the spoken word.

Another important finding is that the response to painful stimulus may be affected by partial or complete paralysis or sensory loss of one half of the body. This is a very important observation to chart, particularly if there is a difference of response between the two sides of the body, and if this difference appears to be increasing. This obviously indicates some kind of progressively increasing damage to one side of the brain.

There are two main reasons for an altered state of consciousness following a head injury. Firstly, there may be widespread brain damage involving the cerebral hemispheres and the brain-stem, sustained at the time of the accident. This may be associated with multiple small haemorrhages and tearing of the nerve fibres in the white matter, lesions which are often seen in the brains of patients who die from head injuries. Secondly (and very important in practice), there may be a deepening state of unconsciousness due to compression of the upper brain-stem by an expanding lesion, usually a clot (*haematoma*) over the surface of the brain (Figure 37).

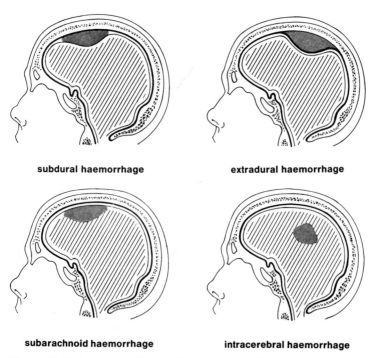

subdural haemorrhage

extradural haemorrhage

subarachnoid haemorrhage

intracerebral haemorrhage

Figure 37 Various types of haemorrhage associated with head injury

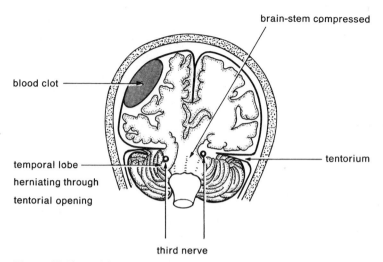

Figure 38 Tentorial herniation

As the clot pushes the cerebral hemisphere to the opposite side and downward, the temporal lobe presses the brain-stem against the tough connective tissue membrane (the *tentorium*) which lies below the temporal lobe and above the cerebellum. This is known as *tentorial herniation* (Figure 38) of the temporal lobe. The upper part of the brain-stem, which normally lies in the middle of the tentorial opening, contains a group of nerve cells called the *reticular formation* which is concerned in a complex way with consciousness. Disturbances in this area may result in coma and eventually death. The other structure which lies closely related to the temporal lobe and the edge of the tentorium is the third (oculomotor) nerve, which can also become compressed. This will result in drooping of the eye-lid (ptosis) and dilatation of the pupil (mydriasis), which then reacts less briskly to a shining light. This is the reason why the size and light reaction of the two pupils are always charted on a head-injuries chart. Compression of the brain-stem also affects the pulse rate, which becomes slower, and the respirations, which become slower and less regular. Ultimately, all the structures in the brain-stem can become involved and a state of *decerebrate rigidity* is produced with the patient's limbs, head and neck stiffly extended while both pupils are dilated and unresponsive to light.

Open and closed injuries

Head injuries can be divided into *open* or *closed* injuries (Figure 39). In open injuries, there is damage to the bones of the skull so that the meninges or the brain becomes exposed, even if only partially. The exposure need not be to the outside; a fracture of the bones of the paranasal sinuses, which are full of air, will result in an open injury. A closed head injury is one where there is no break of the brain coverings, so that the organ remains protected.

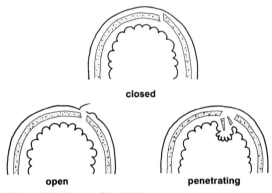

Figure 39 Types of head injury

Fracture of bones may result in penetration of the brain by bone particles. This kind of penetrating brain injury can also occur if the penetration comes from a bullet or particles of clothing, such as a hat. Fracture of the frontal bone and tearing of the dura may give rise to leakage of the cerebrospinal fluid into the frontal sinus and thence to the nose, known as *C S F rhinorrhoea*. Open (particularly if they are also penetrating) head injuries are liable to infection by organisms. This does not occur in closed head injuries, which are, however, liable to the development of an expanding blood clot or haematoma. It is important to realize that the severity of a head injury depends on the amount of brain damage it has caused, and is often quite unrelated to the damage to the skull bones. Thus, severe brain damage may occur without any evidence of skull fracture and, equally, a fractured skull may not be accompanied by a significant degree of brain damage.

Apart from the immediate brain damage, the main complications of a head injury are haemorrhage, infection and epilepsy.

Brain haemorrhage
Extradural haematoma

The blood clot arises from a rupture of one of the arteries outside the dura mater, especially the middle meningeal artery. This injury is usually associated with a fracture of the skull. Typically, immediately after the injury, the patient may not be unconscious at all or, if unconscious, then only for a short time. Then, after a so-called *lucid interval*, there is rapid diminution of consciousness and evidence of tentorial herniation as described above.

Extradural haematoma is a condition of extreme importance and urgency, and immediate neurosurgical treatment is required. Otherwise, death results from compression of the brain-stem. It is because of the existence of this condition that head-injury patients are kept under such careful observation in hospital. The neurosurgical treatment consists of boring holes (*burr-holes*) in the skull bones and removing the blood clot through these. The bleeding artery is tied off at the same time. If the procedure is carried out in time, there may be no ill effects at all on recovery.

Subdural haematoma

Here, the bleeding comes from small veins lying between the dura and the brain. It is therefore a less acute condition than an extradural haematoma, as the pressure in the veins is much less than that in arteries. Typically, therefore, a subdural haematoma develops slowly and shows itself days, weeks or even months after a head injury, presenting as a *space-occupying lesion*, which may be mistaken for a tumour or an abscess. There may not even be a clear history of head injury in the past. The blood clot, developing slowly, is surrounded by a connective tissue membrane. The symptoms and signs are those of rising intracranial pressure, vomiting and papilloedema, drowsiness which may fluctuate from day to day, (or even hour to hour) and weakness, usually a hemiplegia, on the side opposite to the blood clot. The haematoma can be outlined by an arteriogram and evacuated by a neurosurgical operation.

Infection

Infection of the brain and meninges can occur in open head injuries. The infected material enters either from outside the skull or from within one of the paranasal sinuses, depending on the site of the fracture. Patients with CSF rhinorrhoea are particularly liable to develop this complication as they obviously have an opening allowing access to infecting organisms. Infection may result in the development of either meningitis or cerebral abscess and very occasionally the development of osteomyelitis of bone. Antibiotics are essential in the treatment, and surgical procedures may be necessary to evacuate an abscess, remove infected material from the cranium and repair the dura.

Epilepsy

Epilepsy may occur immediately after a head injury and not recur later, or occasionally it may appear months or years afterwards. It is more likely to occur if there has been a depressed fracture of the skull, and particularly if the brain has been penetrated and infected. Treatment consists of the administration of anticonvulsant drugs (see p. 95), but occasionally a scar can be removed from the brain if it is a site which is surgically accessible and unlikely to result in significant post-operative neurological damage such as hemiplegia or dysphasia.

Post-traumatic syndrome

Occasionally, following a head injury, the patient may complain for weeks or months of a combination of symptoms such as headache, giddiness, irritability, depression, poor memory and difficulty in concentration. Although in some cases this may be perpetuated by medico-legal proceedings involving compensation, in most cases it is likely that, at least initially, there is some disturbance of the balance mechanism in the brain-stem or in the inner ear. This results in giddiness, often related to movement of the head, and also a greater or lesser degree of depression causing a vicious circle of tension headache and difficulty in concentration, followed by further anxiety and depression.

In most of these patients, reassurance coupled with the appropriate tranquillizers and antidepressants results in complete relief of the symptoms.

Summary of nursing points

With the increasing number of road traffic accidents, the incidence of head injury is also higher. The patient may be admitted to hospital either for observation or for more detailed surgical treatment, depending on the extent of the injury. The nurse must maintain observations of the level of consciousness, pupil reaction, pulse rate and volume, blood pressure, the rate and depth of breathing and also the behaviour pattern of the patient. Observations must be made of all the orifices of the head (the ear, the nose and the mouth) for signs of bleeding or CSF, which may show as a watery discharge. If a discharge is noticed, it must be reported immediately so that prompt remedial treatment can be initiated.

The nursing care of the patient is vital in ensuring his uneventful recovery. Artificial ventilation may sometimes be indicated to augment respiratory effort. A tracheostomy may be performed, to reduce dead space and to effect pharyngo-tracheal toilet. The patient must be nursed in a semiprone position, and a clear airway must be maintained. The patient should be turned at regular intervals (usually every two hours), and the skin should be kept clean and dry. When extensive paralysis is present and there is resulting loss of muscular activity and a subsequent reduction in heat production, it is necessary to ensure constant body temperature. If the patient is being artificially fed with a nasogastric tube, care must be taken to ensure that the fluid does not enter the air passages.

Chapter 6

Infections of the nervous system

The nervous system may become infected with a variety of living organisms, varying in size from large parasites, such as the malarial parasite or certain worms, down to fungi, bacteria and viruses. Infection gives rise to an inflammatory reaction in the tissues involved. This consists of an increase in the size of the blood vessels (*vasodilatation*), and an outpouring of white blood cells and fluid from the capillaries, so that there is local swelling and pus formation. Pus consists of a mixture of white blood cells (mainly polymorphonuclear leucocytes), dead tissue, infecting organisms and tissue fluid. Inflammation of the brain itself is known as *encephalitis*, inflammation of the spinal cord as *myelitis* and inflammation of the meninges as *meningitis*. There may also be combinations of these diseases, such as encephalomyelitis or meningoencephalitis. When a collection of pus becomes encapsulated, that is, surrounded by a capsule of connective tissue, it is known as an abscess. Depending on the rapidity of onset and progression, infective conditions may be divided into *acute*, *subacute* and *chronic*. Some infections are self-limiting – they stop progressing without any specific treatment. Others respond to appropriate chemicals (*chemotherapeutic agents*), whilst some, such as the viruses, have no specific treatment as yet.

Acute pyogenic meningitis

Pyogenic (purulent or pus-producing) *meningitis* is usually caused by bacteria such as meningococci, pneumococci, staphylococci or *Haemophilus influenzae*. The cerebrospinal fluid (CSF) is cloudy and contains many organisms and white blood cells, mainly polymorphonuclear leucocytes. The organisms may enter the subarachnoid space from the nose and pharynx via the blood stream or, less commonly, after a head injury by penetration through infected bone, from the mastoid cavity or the air sinuses.

The onset is sudden with headache, vomiting, fever and photophobia (dislike of bright light). Inflammation of the meninges gives rise to a stiff neck with resistance to flexion and a positive *Kernig's sign* (Figure 40). This means that the patient feels pain if the knee is straightened when the hip is flexed. The doctor will perform a lumbar puncture (LP) so that a specimen of CSF can be examined (Figure 41). In the CSF there will be many pus cells (white blood cells) and also bacteria which can be seen under the microscope and grown on a special medium; the sugar level is

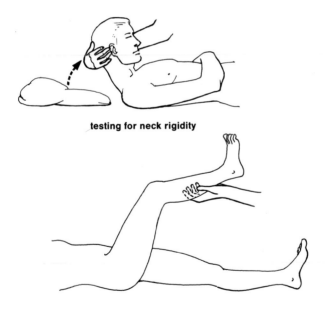

testing for neck rigidity

testing for Kernig's sign

Figure 40 Tests for meningitis

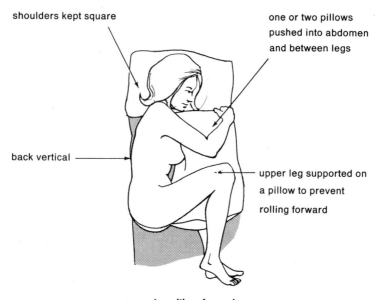

shoulders kept square

one or two pillows pushed into abdomen and between legs

back vertical

upper leg supported on a pillow to prevent rolling forward

correct position, from above

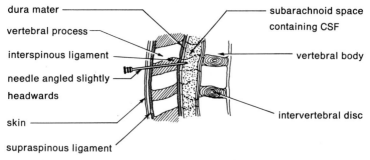

dura mater

subarachnoid space containing CSF

vertebral process

interspinous ligament

vertebral body

needle angled slightly headwards

skin

intervertebral disc

supraspinous ligament

correct insertion of needle

Figure 41 Lumbar puncture

reduced and protein level usually raised. As soon as the diagnosis has been made, treatment is started, usually by giving a mixture of antibiotics. Therapy may be modified when the exact nature of the organism causing the meningitis is known, which should be within 24 hours. The antibiotics are given *parenterally* (intramuscularly or intravenously), and initially sometimes *intrathecally* (into the CSF at the end of the lumbar puncture). Whatever antibiotics are used in this way, it is essential to remember that the intrathecal dose is much less than the intramuscular (usually 10 000 to 20 000 units of penicillin). An excessive dose given intrathecally will result in permanent damage to the nervous system or even the death of the patient – mistakes of this kind are made every year, and the careful nurse can help to prevent them.

Aseptic meningitis

This is the name given to acute meningitis in which no bacteria can be found at any stage. It may occur during the course of a virus infection such as mumps or glandular fever. It may also follow inoculations or infections such as chickenpox, when it is thought to be some kind of allergic reaction rather than a direct infection of the CSF with the virus. It is usually much less severe than a pyogenic bacterial meningitis and resolves spontaneously in the absence of any specific treatment. The CSF contains an increased number of cells, mainly lymphocytes, normal sugar level and only slightly raised protein.

Tuberculosis of the nervous system

Although now much less common, tuberculosis still occurs both in developed and developing countries. It may involve the nervous system and produce severe damage or death unless it is treated early and adequately. Tuberculosis of the nervous system is always secondary to a tuberculous infection elsewhere (usually in the lung).

A small tuberculous focus (*tuberculoma*), in the meninges or within the brain substance, ruptures into the CSF giving rise to meningitis. This usually produces subacute or even chronic symptoms, with a history of many days duration of general malaise, loss of appetite, recurring headaches and slight fever, later followed by vomiting, drowsiness and impaired consciousness, progressing if untreated to coma or death. There may be various kinds of cranial nerve palsies, particularly of the oculomotor nerves with resultant squint and double vision. The pus in the subarachnoid space may become organized into scar tissue, blocking the circulation of CSF by obstructing the outlets from the ventricles. This may rise to ventricular dilatation (*hydrocephalus*) and to spinal-cord compression, causing paralysis of the limbs and sensory loss below the level of the constriction.

The diagnosis of tuberculous meningitis is made by finding tubercle bacilli in the CSF, though this may require the examination of several

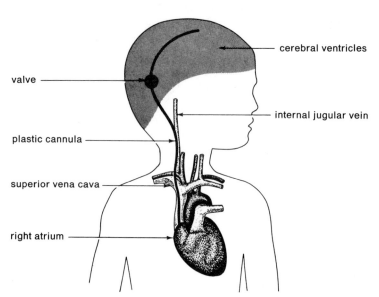

Figure 42 Treatment of hydrocephalus by relieving the tension created by the distension of the cerebral ventricles. The special valve permits fluid to pass from the cerebral ventricles to the atrium

specimens and perhaps culturing the CSF on a special bacteriological medium. Unfortunately, culture takes up to three weeks. The CSF contains an increased number of cells, mainly lymphocytes, the sugar level is low and protein high. In cases where the diagnosis is suspected very strongly, as well as in those where it is confirmed early on, treatment with the anti-tuberculous drugs is started immediately. It is usual to begin with *streptomycin* intramuscularly and *para-aminosalicylic acid* (PAS) and *isonicotinic acid hydrazide* (INAH) by mouth. This combination prevents the bacillus from developing resistance to any of the three drugs. Treatment with at least two drugs may have to be continued for a period of up to two years. An important side-effect of long-term treatment with streptomycin is the development of deafness and loss of balance due to damage to the eighth nerve. If obstruction of ventricles and hydrocephalus develops, the patient, who up till now has been improving, develops headache, confusion and increasing drowsiness. The presence of hydrocephalus is confirmed by appropriate neuroradiological investigation such as air-encephalography (see p. 61) or ventriculography.

In order to relieve the hydrocephalus, the neurosurgeon has to carry out a shunt operation diverting the CSF from the ventricles either to the subarachnoid space or directly into the venous system in the neck; he does this by connecting the ventricles to the jugular vein through a tube with a one-way valve (Figure 42). This valve allows the CSF to pass downwards, but prevents the blood from the veins from entering the ventricles.

Tuberculosis may also involve the spine. It can give rise to infection of one or several vertebrae, producing pain and gradual vertebral collapse. This condition is known as *Pott's disease of the spine*. The spinal deformity and the presence of tuberculous pus under tension may cause compression of the spinal cord and *Pott's paraplegia*. In addition to treatment with antibiotics, appropriate orthopaedic procedures are required to eradicate the disease and stabilize the spine.

Cerebral abscess

This may be caused by infection spreading directly from suppurative middle-ear disease or mastoiditis, from chronic or acute sinusitis, or by the blood stream from such sources as a lung abscess, osteomyelitis (bone infection) or subacute bacterial endocarditis (infection of the heart valves). The symptoms of the disorder are broadly similar to those of any space-occupying lesion such as cerebral tumour (see p. 56), as well as those of inflammation – fever and stiff neck. Treatment consists of the administration of the appropriate antibiotics and the evacuation of pus from the abscess by the neurosurgeon.

Viral encephalitis

This condition, which is not uncommon, varies in severity. In most cases no specific virus can ever be named as being responsible even after very full investigation. It can be caused by such viruses as *Herpes simplex* (which is the cause of the common cold sore around the lips), *Herpes zoster* (shingles) and Japanese B. It may be spread by mosquito bites, or by direct contact from person to person. Its symptoms may be very mild, such as slight headache and fever, or more severe and rapidly fatal with increasing headache, confusion and coma. The CSF may contain an increased number of white cells, mainly lymphocytes. A variety of preparations have been used in its treatment, as reliable antiviral drugs do not as yet exist. Adrenal cortical steroids or ACTH are sometimes given as they tend to reduce brain swelling and may relieve some of the symptoms.

Viral myelitis

Poliomyelitis virus specifically invades the anterior horn cells of the spinal cord and the corresponding motor neurones in the brain-stem. It enters the nervous system via the blood stream (*viraemia*) after initial infection of the gastrointestinal tract through direct contamination of food with faecal material from already-infected persons. Only a small proportion, perhaps 10 per cent, of infected persons develop evidence of CNS involvement and this, in the majority of patients, consists of a mild meningitis with fever, headache, a slightly stiff neck and muscle pains. Only about 10 per cent of these patients develop evidence of involvement of the motor neurones – that is, varying degrees of paralysis. Again, in the majority of patients, the paralysis is mild and transient.

Fortunately, now that effective inoculation against poliomyelitis exists, it is a rare condition but, in the days of epidemics, its effects were often crippling or fatal. When the brain-stem is involved, paralysis of the muscles of respiration and of swallowing results. This serious condition requires artificial ventilation and tube feeding. Usually these patients also recover a good deal of function within a few weeks, though some have to adapt themselves to life-long tracheostomy and artificial ventilation.

Parasitic infections

The most common of these is *malaria*. The malarial parasite is transmitted by a mosquito bite and, in people not taking anti-malarial drugs, it passes in the blood to the liver and later throughout the body. It may block the cerebral capillaries, producing cerebral malaria which results, if untreated, in deepening coma and death. Nowadays, with the increasing ease of air travel, it is important to be aware of such diseases, which can be contracted during even a short stay in the transit lounge of an airport unless anti-malarial prophylactic drugs are taken. Treatment consists primarily of intravenous quinine or chloroquinine and a variety of other supportive measures.

Sleeping sickness (*trypanosomiasis*), transmitted from infected cattle by the tsetse fly, is another potentially fatal infection of the brain. It is usually a chronic illness with headache, increasing lethargy and coma occurring if the disease is untreated. There is also fever and enlargement of the lymph glands and spleen.

Cysticercosis is caused by larvae of the human tapeworm, which invade brain and muscle. Cysts in muscle may calcify but do no harm, whereas in the brain they may cause epilepsy or raised intracranial pressure, due to obstruction of the flow of CSF.

Trichiniasis (trichinosis) is caused by eating undercooked pork containing a parasite which can produce an encephalitis and myositis (inflammation of muscles), with muscle pains, swelling and weakness.

Hydatid cysts may occur in the brain. They are formed by the parasite *Echinococcus granulosus*, which is harboured by sheep. This condition is not uncommon in countries with large sheep populations such as parts of Wales, the Middle East, Australia and New Zealand. It gives rise to symptoms and signs of a space-occupying intracranial lesion and the brain cysts may have to be removed surgically.

Neurosyphilis

This is a rare disease today. The first stage is the infection of the genital organs with the spirochaete *Treponema pallidum*. The second stage occurs some weeks or months later and is characterized by fever, skin rashes and very occasionally meningitis.

The tertiary stage may not occur until some years later. The effects on the central nervous system are due to the inflammation of the small arteries – usually those passing through the meninges and entering the brain and spinal cord. This form is known as *meningovascular syphilis*. The symptoms and signs are those of cerebral infarction secondary to the arteritis. Thus, there may be a variety of 'stroke' resulting in hemiplegia, but often the arteries involved may be those supplying an individual cranial nerve, in which case an isolated cranial nerve palsy results. Alternatively, if the artery involved supplies the spinal cord, there may be sudden onset of a transverse cord lesion or myelitis with loss of power and sensation below the level of the lesion.

The fourth stage, which may occur without any preceding manifestations of neurosyphilis, has one of two forms. One is *tabes dorsalis* in which the destruction of the sensory ganglia occurs and results in the loss of position-sense in the limbs and loss of pain, temperature and touch sensation. In addition to the sensory loss, involvement of the dorsal root ganglion cells often gives rise to recurrent excruciating spontaneous pains in any part of the body. As they are only momentary they are known as lightning pains. If they occur in the abdomen they may lead to a mistaken diagnosis of some intra-abdominal condition such as renal colic or appendicitis.

The other form is known as *general paralysis of the insane* (GPI). It is caused by progressive loss of neurones in the cerebral cortex, resulting in convulsions, intellectual deterioration (*dementia*) and the development of a generalized upper motor neurone paralysis.

In many patients with neurosyphilis, there is an abnormality of the pupils known as the *Argyll–Robertson pupils.* Such pupils are small, irregular, and do not react (constrict) to light, but do react when looking very closely at an object (accommodation). This abnormality is a useful sign of neurosyphilis in patients who may have none of the other features of this condition.

The diagnosis of syphilis is confirmed by a variety of blood tests. The oldest is the *Wasserman reaction* (WR). Other blood tests have been developed in recent years. The *treponema pallidum immobilization* (TPI) test is also very helpful. These tests are also often positive in the CSF of patients with neurosyphilis. Care is needed in the interpretation of any test for VD. A positive WR test does *not* always mean that the patient has the disease, for it may be positive during pregnancy, following glandular fever and always in yaws, a skin infection common in certain tropical countries. Treatment of neurosyphilis consists of the administration of penicillin or other appropriate antibiotics.

Summary of nursing points

The common inflammatory conditions of the nervous system include meningitis and encephalitis. The causes include parasites, worms, fungi, bacteria and viruses, while the sources include systemic infections, mastoiditis, chronic sinusitis, bacterial endocarditis and osteomyelitis. The nurse should understand the principles of pathology, together with its clinical manifestations, investigations, methods of prevention, complications and treatment. She should also be aware of the real danger of cross-infection and therefore take the necessary precautions by barrier nursing the patient. She must be particularly careful of all discharge from all orifices, and ensure that it is disposed of without endangering other patients.

Observations must be made of the temperature, pulse, respiration and blood pressure, fluid balance, level of consciousness and any change in behaviour. Any abnormalities must be noted and reported promptly, so that adjustments can be made as indicated. Drugs must be given as prescribed, and their effects noted and reported.

Chapter 7

Disorders of peripheral nerves and muscles

The peripheral nerves consist of a mixture of motor, sensory and autonomic nerve fibres. The cell body (neurone) of the motor fibre lies in the anterior horn of the spinal cord (Figure 43), that of the sensory fibre lies in the dorsal root ganglion just outside the spinal cord, and the sympathetic (thoraco-lumbar) and parasympathetic (cranio-sacral) ganglia contain the autonomic neurones. Disorders of the motor fibres of peripheral nerves produce weakness, wasting and loss of tendon reflexes. Those involving the sensory fibres produce impairment or complete loss of sensation in the areas of the skin and in the joints supplied by the particular nerve. There may also be pins-and-needles or tingling sensations (*paraesthesiae*). Involvement of the autonomic nerve fibres may produce impairment of sweating and alterations in the pupil of the eye, disturbances of bladder and sex function and of blood pressure control.

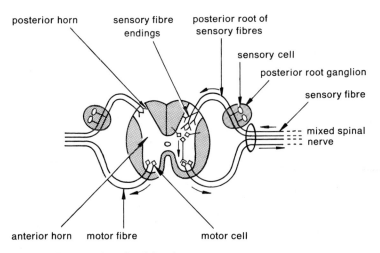

Figure 43 Formation of peripheral nerves

Peripheral nerve disorders may involve the motor, sensory and autonomic nerve fibres to a varying extent. A generalized involvement of many or all of the peripheral nerves is termed a peripheral neuritis (*neuropathy*). Lesions may also affect only one nerve, for instance where there is damage through injury or from chronic pressure, as on the median nerve at the wrist.

Infective polyneuritis

Over the whole world the most common infection causing peripheral neuritis is leprosy. The leprosy bacillus (*Mycobacterium leprae*), is probably infective if exposure to it occurs over a period of years. It multiplies in the *Schwann cells* (the supporting cells surrounding the nerve axons), and causes either a localized or a generalized neuritis with motor and sensory involvement. Because the disease is chronic, deformities in the limbs, and particularly the hands and feet, may develop due to loss of muscle power and of sensation. Leprosy can now be arrested and even cured by the administration of appropriate drugs. The deformities resulting from the chronic peripheral neuritis can often be relieved by orthopaedic and plastic reconstructive surgery.

Another infection causing peripheral neuritis, now fortunately very uncommon because of effective immunization, is diphtheria. In diphtheria the toxin produced by the bacillus damages peripheral nerves but this may not show itself for some weeks after the throat infection. Usually the first symptom is palatal paralysis, followed by paralysis of accommodation of the eye muscles (failure to constrict the pupil when looking at near objects) and finally weakness and sensory disturbance in the limbs. Recovery takes place spontaneously.

Acute infective polyneuritis (the *Guillain–Barré syndrome*) is thought to be some kind of allergic reaction to a variety of causes such as virus infections, vaccination or immunization. The disease usually begins with numbness and tingling in the feet and hands, followed within a day or two by increasing weakness of the limbs or even of the muscles of swallowing and respiration. Ultimate recovery is likely with gradual return of the lost power and sensation but, in severely paralysed patients, this may take weeks or months. If the muscles of swallowing and respiration are involved, artificial respiration through a tracheostomy and nasal feeding are required. In some patients ACTH or cortisone given in the early stages may reduce the severity of the developing weakness.

Toxic and deficiency neuropathies

Many drugs used in medicine, as well as certain industrial and naturally occurring substances, can damage peripheral nerves. INAH used in the treatment of tuberculosis and nitrofurantoin used in urinary tract infections are examples of the former. Heavy metals, such as lead, and certain insecticides containing arsenic and other substances may be inhaled or ingested in small amounts over long periods by people working with them, and so produce chronic peripheral neuritis.

Deficiencies of certain vitamins, particularly B_1 (*thiamine*) and B_{12} (*cyanocobalamine*) may cause peripheral neuritis. Thiamine deficiency is usually due to poor diet and causes the tropical disease *beriberi*, in which peripheral neuritis may be accompanied by heart failure. Thiamine deficiency may also be a contributory cause of the neuropathy seen in chronic alcoholics. It is associated with poor diet and perhaps interference by alcohol with absorption and metabolism of the vitamin.

Vitamin B_{12} deficiency usually gives rise to *pernicious anaemia*. There is failure to absorb the vitamin from the gastrointestinal tract because of the absence of a substance known as the *intrinsic factor* in the stomach wall. The deficiency may cause damage to the spinal cord and peripheral nerves (*subacute combined degeneration*); there may be optic-nerve atrophy with blindness, and also occasionally dementia. The condition can be completely reversed if treated early by the regular administration of vitamin B_{12} injections.

Metabolic neuropathy

The most common of these is the neuropathy of *diabetes mellitus*. It usually produces only a mild sensory disturbance. However, it may occasionally produce marked muscle weakness, which may be patchy and involve only certain muscles in one limb (*diabetic amyotrophy*), probably due to impaired blood supply to individual peripheral nerves because of the obstruction of the small arteries supplying them. Diabetic neuropathy tends to occur in patients with long-standing diabetes and shows some response to strict control of the blood-sugar level with diet, insulin or appropriate oral anti-diabetic drugs. Diabetic neuropathy affecting the feet is often associated with diabetic vascular disease and the likely occurrence of ulcers on toes and feet in such patients calls for special care of feet and nails.

Very rarely, neuropathy may be due to one of the groups of disorders known as the *porphyrias*. There may be associated mental confusion made worse by barbiturate sleeping tablets or anaesthetic. Characteristically, the patient's urine turns dark on standing.

Isolated peripheral nerve lesions

These usually occur as a result of trauma such as gunshot wounds, lacerations or motor accidents. If a nerve has been completely severed, the part beyond the cut degenerates completely while nerve fibres sprout from the near end of the cut nerve and (as long as they are able to find it) grow down the nerve sheath of the already degenerated nerve at the rate of about 1–2 mm a day. In order to aid the nerve fibres in finding the end of the degenerated nerve, it is important to excise any scar tissue and to suture the two ends.

One nerve which unfortunately is particularly liable to damage by an inadvertent deep intramuscular injection is the sciatic nerve in the muscles of the buttock. It is essential when giving such an injection to keep to the

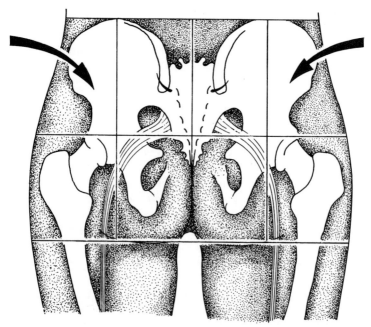

Figure 44 The correct place to give an injection in the buttock; the upper outer quandrants are used to avoid the sciatic nerve and the bony points

upper outer quadrant of the buttock which is well clear of the nerve (Figure 44).

Certain peripheral nerves may become damaged because they are very superficially placed under the skin and may be pressed on to the underlying bone. This occurs sometimes with the ulnar nerve (Figure 45) as it passes on the medial side of the elbow joint in what is known as the groove on the olecranon part of the humerus. It is likely to happen to bedridden or

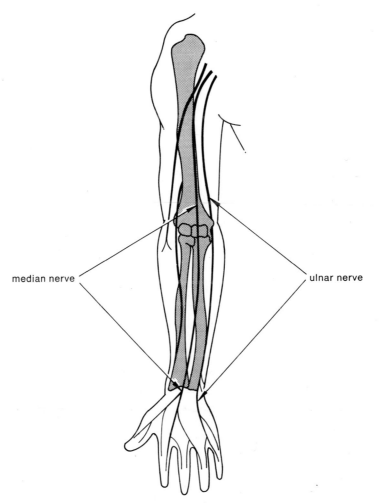

median nerve

ulnar nerve

Figure 45 The median and ulnar nerves in the arm

chair-ridden patients, who may spend much time leaning on their elbows, and also to patients with elbow joints deformed from arthritis. Compression of the ulnar nerve produces tingling and sensory impairment in the little and ring fingers and corresponding part of the hand, and weakness of the small hand muscles. It is relieved by an operation in which the nerve is transposed from the back to the front of the elbow giving it more protection from repeated pressure.

The common peroneal nerve may be compressed behind the head of the fibula in bedridden patients who have lost weight, producing *foot drop* (weakness of upward extension of the foot). This condition usually recovers spontaneously.

Carpal tunnel syndrome

This is a common condition, especially in middle-aged women. The median nerve, which supplies the muscles of the thumb, passes from the forearm into the hand through a tunnel-like structure between the carpal bone at the wrist and a tough connective tissue band, the *flexor retinaculum* (Figure 46). In this tunnel, the nerve lies close to the tendons of the flexor muscles passing to the fingers and thumb. If the contents of the carpal tunnel swell up even slightly, the median nerve becomes compressed. Such a swelling may occur during pregnancy (when it is part of a generalized oedema), in hypothyroidism (*myxoedema*), in obese women, and also if the flexor tendons become inflamed through unaccustomed excessive exercise – for instance, after painting and decorating, or in mothers of newborn children after having to wash and wring out nappies. Occasionally no obvious cause for the development of this condition exists.

The symptoms consist of unpleasant tingling, pins-and-needles and numbness in the thumb, index and middle fingers, pain in the wrist and sometimes in the whole arm, and weakness and wasting of the muscles at the base of the thumb (*the thenar eminence*). The definitive treatment is surgical: the division at operation of the flexor retinaculum, which allows more room for the contents of the carpal tunnel. Sometimes relief is obtained either by injecting hydrocortisone into the carpal tunnel, so diminishing the oedema and inflammation, or by providing the patient with a splint for the wrist to wear by day and night.

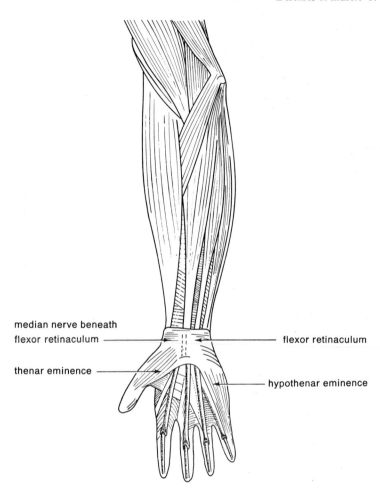

Figure 46 The median nerve at the wrist

Diseases of muscle

Muscles can be divided according to their appearance under the miscroscope into *striated* and *smooth* (Figure 47). Striated muscles are those which are responsible for skeletal movements. Smooth muscle is present in the walls of visceral structures such as the gastrointestinal

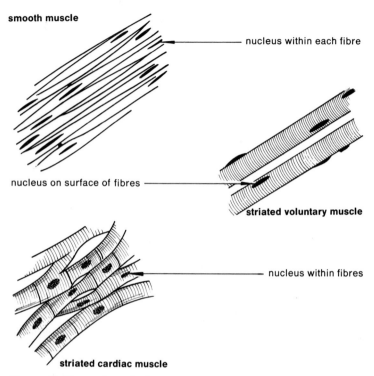

Figure 47 Types of muscle tissue

tract, the ureters, the bladder, the uterus and also the blood vessels. Striated muscle receives its motor nerve supply from motor neurones in the brain-stem and spinal cord. Smooth muscle is innervated by autonomic nerve fibres. *Cardiac muscle* is sometimes known as mixed as it has some properties of striated and some of smooth muscle.

Muscle disorders are of two main types, inherited and acquired. The inherited muscle disorders (*muscular dystrophies*) have descriptive names depending largely on the distribution of the muscle weakness and wasting. *Pseudohypertrophic muscular dystrophy* is named after the appearance of apparently enlarged calves of the affected male children. This is due to an excessive amount of fatty and connective tissue in place of muscle fibres, hence, 'pseudohypertrophy'. The disease affects some of the male children of mothers who carry the abnormal gene responsible for the disease. Children with this disorder develop weakness in the third or fourth year of life and deteriorate over the course of the next ten years, ultimately dying when the respiratory muscles become paralysed.

Another kind of muscular dystrophy which affects the facial, shoulder and pelvic muscles is known as the *facio-scapulo-humeral* type. It usually begins in early adult life and its progress is much slower so that patients, though disabled, may survive into late adult life. The *limb girdle dystrophies* affect particularly the shoulder and pelvic girdle muscles.

A condition known as *dystrophia myotonica* is a muscular dystrophy in which, in addition to weakness (usually beginning in adult life and progressing slowly), certain muscles cannot relax after a contraction (*myotonia*). Typically, the hands are involved and the patient is unable to release his grip so readily. Patients may also develop cataracts, frontal baldness and testicular or ovarian atrophy.

There is unfortunately no cure for any of the muscular dystrophies. Myotonia is relieved by a variety of drugs such as quinine and procaine amide. An important aspect of these disorders is the detection of carriers of the abnormal gene, who may themselves be unaffected. Methods used consist of the measurement of the blood levels of certain blood enzymes (those concerned with muscle metabolism) and electrical studies on muscles (*electromyography*). Certain tests are also being developed which may enable the diagnosis to be made by examining the amniotic fluid obtained from the uterus of pregnant women.

Acquired muscle disorders or myopathies are also characterized by the development of progressive muscle weakness and wasting. *Polymyositis* (inflammation of muscles) may respond to steroids. Diseases of endocrine glands such as hyperthyroidism, hyperparathyroidism and oversecretion of adrenal hormones (Cushing's disease) may produce metabolic myopathy.

Myasthenia gravis

This disease is due to the failure of correct transmission of nerve impulses from the nerve endings to the muscle fibres at the *neuromuscular junction*. Our nerve endings release a substance known as *acetylcholine* which is responsible for the contraction of muscle fibres, and an adequate concentration of this chemical is not achieved in myasthenia gravis.

The disorder may involve only certain muscles, commonly those concerned with eye movements, so that there is drooping of the lids and *diplopia* (double vision). The muscles of swallowing and of respiration and those of the limbs may also be involved. Treatment consists of administering cholinesterase inhibitors, which prevent the acetylcholine released at the neuromuscular junction from being destroyed by another substance known as *cholinesterase*. The drug used most commonly is *prostigmine* (neostigmine), which has to be given at frequent intervals and is usually very effective. Occasionally overdosage with one of the cholinesterase inhibitors may result in increasing weakness, eventually leading even to respiratory paralysis. Once this has been taken care of by applying artificial ventilation using some form of a respirator, special tests will show whether this increased weakness is due to insufficiency (*myasthenic crisis*) or excess (*cholinergic crisis*) of the drug. A small proportion of patients with myasthenia gravis may have a tumour in the thymus gland and this requires surgical removal though this has little effect on their myasthenia. In some other patients the removal of an apparently normal thymus gland can diminish the symptoms of myasthenia.

Summary of nursing points

The nurse should be familiar with the main disorders of the peripheral nerves. She should understand the clinical manifestations, investigations, treatment and nursing management of infective polyneuritis, toxic and metabolic neuropathy, such as diabetes mellitus and vitamin deficiencies, together with the muscular dystrophies. She must be fully aware of the serious effects of the conditions on the patient, not only the physical aspects, but also the social and emotional ones.

The care of the patient makes many demands on the nurse. If respiratory distress occurs, tracheostomy and artificial ventilation may be indicated. Affected limbs may have to be supported, using sorbo pads and other devices. To prevent damage to the skin, mouth and eyes, regular toilet must be carried out. This is particularly important in peripheral neuritis.

The nurse must observe the patient carefully and constantly for signs of extension of the disease process, such as paralysis. She must report and record any change.

The patient must be constantly assisted in his rehabilitation – physically, socially and emotionally.

Chapter 8

Paroxysmal disorders

Paroxysmal disorders are those in which there are short-lived symptoms, usually of sudden onset. These may consist of a disturbance of consciousness, or attacks of headache or other pain, or of giddiness. The diagnosis of the cause of attacks of loss of consciousness is almost always based on the history of the symptoms preceding the event, and on the description of the patient's behaviour whilst unconscious. Among the possible causes of loss of consciousness are epilepsy, syncope (fainting) and hypoglycaemic attacks.

A trained observer, such as the nurse or the doctor, can provide particularly useful information, such as whether or not there was any warning or any symptoms before the patient passed out, and whether the patient was unconscious all the time or responded in some way to command. An accurate description of the attack is essential, including a description of any movements. Other points to be noted are: which side of the body is affected, whether the head was turned to one side or the other, whether there was any incontinence or tongue-biting, whether the pulse rate was very slow, very fast or irregular, the patient's colour at different stages, and whether he was sweating excessively. After the attack, it should be noted whether the patient was confused and if there was any localized paralysis of the limbs. A nurse may also be in a position to examine a patient during or immediately after an attack and determine whether his plantar responses are flexor or extensor (*Babinski's sign*). Knowledge of this may be very valuable in establishing the diagnosis of the cause of an attack.

Epilepsy

Epilepsy occurs in about one in every two hundred people. It is not a disease in itself, but merely a symptom of an illness, usually of the nervous system but occasionally metabolic or biochemical in nature. An epileptic attack may begin in many different ways and be associated with varied symptoms. In the brain, it begins with the sudden abnormal discharge of electrical waves from a small localized area (*focus*). What happens next depends on where this focus happens to be. If it is in the motor cortex, it results in involuntary jerking of a limb or limbs. If it is in the sensory cortex, the patient experiences paraesthesiae (pins-and-needles or tingling). If it is in the visual cortex, there may be visual hallucinations such as flashing lights or more organized scenes of people or incidents. A typical motor or sensory attack begins in the fingers or a corner of the mouth and spreads up the limb and then into the other one on the same side. This type of attack is known as a *Jacksonian attack*. All these different kinds of symptoms which the patient may experience before losing consciousness are known as the *aura*, and may last up to a minute or two. The symptoms of temporal lobe attacks, caused by a focus in one temporal lobe, are characterized by an abnormal sensation of smell (*olfactory aura*) or of taste and may consist of a transient confusion with purposeless activities such as smacking of lips or repetitive picking (*psychomotor attacks*).

In the most common type of adult epilepsy, an electrical discharge spreads widely throughout the brain so that there is loss of consciousness, usually accompanied by a generalized convulsion. At first the body and limbs become rigid, while the tongue may be bitten and the respirations may contract. This is known as the *tonic phase*, and it may last several seconds. The muscles then relax and contract alternately. This is the *clonic* phase, which may last several minutes. The patient may be incontinent of urine and even of faeces. Afterwards there may be a period of confusion, during which the patient may perform some automatic actions of which he may later have no recollection. Immediately after an attack, the limbs which were particularly severely involved in the convulsive movements may show transient weakness, known as *Todd's paralysis*.

Attacks in which there is loss of consciousness are known as major attacks or *grand mal*. Those in which there is no loss of consciousness are known as minor attacks. Not all major attacks are preceded by an aura or warning symptoms. Sometimes there may be sudden loss of consciousness without any warning, with or without a major convulsion. These attacks without a preceding aura are thought to be due to the electrical discharge arising from the part of the upper brain-stem concerned with consciousness, the reticular formation.

In *petit mal*, a form of minor epilepsy common in children, there is a very sudden and very short-lived disturbance of consciousness. The child stops whatever it is doing and, for a second or two, stares into space. He may not even know that an attack has occurred though, if several occur in quick succession, he may miss part of the conversation or a school lesson. Patients with petit mal may occasionally suffer from *myoclonic jerks*, sudden violent jerking movements of one or both arms. If the legs are involved, there may be a sudden fall without loss of consciousness known as a *drop attack*.

Febrile convulsions are major attacks occurring in children in the first few years of life. They are associated with a high or rising fever, and may occur during such illnesses as tonsillitis, ear infections or pneumonia. Their presence indicates that the child is probably more prone than the average to convulse when under some sort of physical stress, but the majority of those affected do not develop epilepsy in later life. Immediately after a convulsion, treatment should be directed to getting the child's temperature down, by removing its clothes, by turning off all heating, by giving aspirin by mouth and by tepid sponging of the skin.

Causes of epileptic convulsions
Even after a very full investigation, the cause of epileptic convulsions is found in less than half the patients. The condition may be classified into two types: *symptomatic*, where it is a symptom of some established disorder and *idiopathic*, where no cause has been found. Symptomatic causes include a variety of conditions such as brain tumour, brain abscess, inflammation of the brain (encephalitis), syphilis of the brain and some rare conditions of a metabolic nature. Scars in the brain may also give rise to an epileptic focus. Such scars may be the result of birth injury, anoxia and cyanosis at time of birth, or head injury in later life. They may also arise from small healed infarcts – dead tissue in the brain resulting from cerebrovascular disease.

Idiopathic epilepsy, which is more common, may be of two kinds. There are patients in whom the cause cannot be established with certainty at the time of the investigations though it may sometimes become obvious in years to come. There is also a group of patients who may possibly have an inherited predisposition to attacks. Into this particular group fall the attacks of the petit mal variety, the myoclonic jerks and drop attacks, and also those major attacks which occur without an aura preceding them; these are thought to arise from electrical instability of the brain-stem reticular formation. Another way of classifying the epilepsies is into those which arise from the central part of the brain-stem (called *central* or

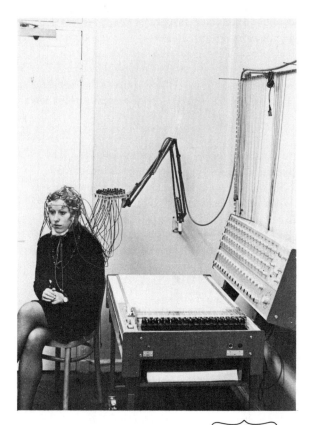

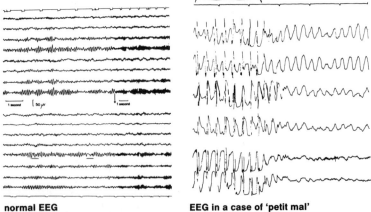

normal EEG

EEG in a case of 'petit mal'

Figure 48 The electroencephalogram (EEG).
In the case of the patient with 'petit mal', the EEG shows a paroxysm of three cycles per second 'spike and wave' activity

generalized) and those which arise from an area of the cortex where there is some focal abnormality (these are called *focal*).

Investigations

In general, certain simple investigations are done in the majority of patients. A skull X-ray may show calcification in a tumour or raised intracranial pressure, and a chest X-ray evidence of carcinoma of the bronchus, a common cause of secondary brain tumour. A blood test for syphilis (the *Wasserman reaction*) should always be carried out. An *electroencephalogram* (EEG) will be done wherever possible in the majority of patients (Figure 48). It may show evidence of a focal abnormality. In children with petit mal it should show a characteristic 'spike and wave' discharge at the rate of 3 to 4 per second.

It must be remembered, however, that even in severe epileptics the EEG record between seizures may be normal and also that about 10 per cent of the normal population may have a mild EEG abnormality. Therefore, the diagnosis of epilepsy should never be based on the EEG record alone. If, for some reason, a brain tumour or some other progressive abnormality is suspected, the patient may need to undergo more specialized neuro-radiological investigations such as a brain scan, an arteriogram or an air-encephalogram.

Treatment

In day-to-day management, the main aim is to enable patients to lead as normal a life as possible. Thus after only one attack it is usual not to place any restrictions on the patient and not to administer anticonvulsant drugs which reduce the possibility of an attack occurring. If fits do recur then a variety of anticonvulsant drugs exist, and these can be administered alone or in various combinations. In the majority of patients, effective control is soon achieved. Patients are advised not to go swimming unless accompanied by a swimmer who will keep them under observation: this usually implies that they should only swim in swimming pools. They should not work at heights or with moving machinery. They should not drive any form of motor vehicle unless the attacks are only nocturnal and are well controlled and if the laws of the land permit them to drive. Children with very infrequent attacks are sometimes allowed to ride bicycles, but not on a public road.

A considerable number of anticonvulsant drugs are available. Petit mal attacks respond well to one or other of the two main groups of specific drugs: the *dione* and the *succinimide* derivatives, the chief example of each being *tridione* and *ethosuccinimide* (Zarontin). In the treatment of major convulsions and of focal attacks, the three most commonly used preparations are *phenobarbitone*, *phenytoin* (Epanutin, Dilantin) and *primidone* (Mysoline). Their main side-effect is drowsiness. Occasionally they may cause an anaemia characterized by the presence of abnormally large (megaloblastic) red cells and even more rarely by bone changes similar to rickets. Phenytoin may also cause hypertrophy of the gums, ataxia, hirsuties (excessive growth of hair) and, rarely, a variety of other complications. One of the most important aspects of drug treatment of epilepsy is that it should never be stopped suddenly as this may result in severe major convulsions. These may also occur if the tablets are frequently forgotten by the patient.

Patients may worry about the effect of epilepsy on the intelligence. Epilepsy in itself does not lead to intellectual deterioration, and many sufferers from the disease (e.g. Socrates, Julius Caesar, Handel, Dante and Dostoyevski) have shown high intelligence. Where the patient's IQ is affected it is probably because the underlying disease causing the epilepsy is also affecting mental function or sometimes because the slowing down is due to the effect of the anti-convulsant treatment – this should then be appropriately adjusted. Not infrequently, patients with epilepsy suffer from anxiety or depression and this kind of reaction may result in impaired performance at school or at work. There is no reason why an epileptic person should not marry and have children, even though some forms of the disease have a greater incidence in other members of the family. The influence of heredity in the epileptic disorders has been greatly over-emphasized in the past. The social aspects of treating the epilepsies are of tremendous importance. Unfortunately, epileptic people have, for centuries, been subjected to all kinds of unfair prejudice. In spite of these potential problems, epileptics should be encouraged to make friends, go in for sports and hobbies and pursue whatever careers they are interested in.

During a major convulsion, the prime consideration is to prevent the patient from causing damage to himself. He should be protected from open or electric fires, sharp furniture or moving machinery. The safest place is probably on the floor. If possible, the collar should be loosened and a soft gag (e.g. a handkerchief) placed between the teeth, but the mouth should not be forced open with any hard object. When the convulsion is over, the patient should be permitted to come round in his own time, allowed to sleep if drowsy and must be kept under observation till he is fully alert and orientated.

Status epilepticus, where convulsions frequently recur without recovery of consciousness between attacks, is a medical emergency requiring urgent treatment. The danger lies in the patient developing brain damage from repeated episodes of disturbed respiration with lack of oxygenation of the brain cells (anoxia). Intramuscular phenobarbitone (100 mg) or paraldehyde (10 ml) or intravenous diazepam (Valium) should be given by injection. The patient should be put on his side in the half-prone position with chest and face facing half-down, but the airway kept clear. This avoids aspiration of secretions or vomit. If the respirations become depressed because of the drugs, then artificial ventilation may be required. If the attack still continues, then intravenous barbiturates may be required after an endotracheal tube has been passed. This situation is best dealt with in an intensive care unit.

A very small proportion of patients whose attacks cannot be controlled adequately by medical means may be considered for surgical treatment. This is feasible if there is only one abnormal area which gives rise to the attacks and if this area is in that part of the brain which, if removed, will not cause significant damage (such as dysphasia or hemiplegia) to the patient on recovery from the operation. Occasionally, scars from head injury or birth injury may be amenable to this kind of radical treatment which has been used particularly for the treatment of some patients with temperal-lobe epilepsy.

Hypoglycaemic attacks

These are rare except in diabetics on insulin. When the level of blood glucose is low or when it is falling rapidly, loss of consciousness may occur. Usually, the onset of unconsciousness is preceded by a period of confusion or even focal symptoms such as weakness or numbness in a limb or half the body, or slurring of speech. Sometimes, the patient may convulse; this is particularly likely in children. Characteristically, there is profuse sweating. The most common cause of a hypoglycaemic attack is an overdose of insulin. Spontaneous hypoglycaemia may occasionally be produced by tumours, usually of the pancreas, which secrete insulin into the blood. If hypoglycaemia is suspected as the cause of such an attack, blood should be taken from the patient for estimation of the glucose level *before* glucose is administered, either by mouth, if the patient is conscious, or intravenously if he is unconscious.

Syncopal attacks (faints)

These are probably the most common cause of loss of consciousness in all age groups. They result from insufficient oxygenation of brain cells because of reduced cerebral circulation. This is caused by a reduced output of blood from the heart because of retention of blood in the veins of the legs and of the abdominal organs. This usually occurs when the patient is standing for a prolonged period in a hot atmosphere or when he suddenly stands up from a lying position, particularly on getting out of bed in the morning. An additional factor which occurs in so-called *micturition syncope* is that, when the bladder is emptied, there is a fall in the blood pressure. Before losing consciousness, there is usually a sensation of faintness or buzzing in the ears, darkening of vision and an alternating feeling of warmth and coldness. The treatment of such an attack is to allow the patient to remain in the horizontal position so that the cerebral circulation can recover. Do *not* fall into the trap of attempting to sit him up.

Some disturbances of the cardiovascular system which interfere with cardiac output of blood may produce syncope by reducing the amount of blood reaching the brain. This can occur with *aortic stenosis* (narrowing of the aortic valve) and with heart block (which results in a very slow heart rate of about 30 to 40 beats per minute). Patients with heart block sometimes have a type of syncope known as a *Stokes–Adams attack*. Typically, the patient goes very pale and collapses unconscious. Seconds later, he usually flushes a bright pink colour as the heart beat recommences, and consciousness is then rapidly regained, though the heart rate remains very slow.

Migraine

This is the name given to a particular kind of headache. Typically, it consists of a unilateral throbbing pain lasting several hours accompanied by nausea, vomiting and photophobia (dislike of bright lights). It may be preceded or accompanied by a visual aura of flashing lights or zig-zag lines, or by blurred vision. This visual aura usually lasts around 30 minutes, unlike the aura of epilepsy which may last only one or two minutes. Sometimes in an attack there may be hemiplegia or hemianaesthesia or dysphasia, which almost always recovers completely. The cause and the mechanism of migraine are unknown. Constriction and dilatation of certain blood vessels in the scalp and within the skull are thought to be concerned with the production of symptoms.

Attacks may occur spontaneously or may be brought on by mental or physical stress or lack of sleep and (in some patients) by certain foods (such as chocolate or oranges) or alcoholic drinks. Treatment of attacks involves rest, preferably in a dark room and the administration of pain-relieving (analgesic) tablets.

Preparations containing the chemical substance *ergotamine* are used both in prevention of attacks and in their treatment. A variety of these exist. Because of nausea and vomiting they may have to be given by intramuscular or subcutaneous injection, as a suppository or as sublingual (under the tongue) tablets. The main serious side-effect of ergotamine preparations is that large doses may constrict the blood vessels in the fingers and toes and result in gangrene, sometimes even of whole limbs. New drugs are constantly being tried for the relief of migraine. Because tension and depression may be a factor responsible for the attacks, treatment with anti-depressants and tranquillizers often has a beneficial effect.

Trigeminal neuralgia (tic douloureux)

In this condition, the patient experiences attacks of pain in the distribution of one of the three branches of the trigeminal nerve (see p. 36). Characteristically, the pain is momentary, stabbing and severe, sometimes like an electric shock. It is brought on by eating, talking, chewing or touching a 'trigger spot' in the affected area. Attacks may last several weeks and then cease spontaneously. The cause of the condition is unknown. Of the various preparations which have been tried over the years to terminate attacks, carbamazepine (Tegretol), taken orally, is the most useful. In very resistant cases, the trigeminal nerve may have to be cut within the skull by the neurosurgeon. Alternatively, the ganglion on the nerve may be destroyed by an injection with alcohol through one of the small openings in the base of the skull. This then results not only in the abolition of the pain but also in permanent numbness of the face and of the cornea so that the patient must thereafter wear protective spectacles to avoid developing a corneal lesion as a result of a foreign body in an anaesthetic eye.

Vertigo and Ménière's disease

Vertigo is a sensation of movement of the environment or of the subject in relation to the environment. It has many causes. Balance is maintained by a complex mechanism which lies in the middle and inner ear, eighth nerve, brain-stem, cerebellum and temporal lobe. It depends also on messages from the neck muscles and the eyes. Balance can therefore be disturbed by disorders involving any of these structures.

Ménière's disease is characterized by progressive deafness, persistent noises in the ear (*tinnitus*) and attacks of vertigo. Its cause is unknown. The severity of any of these three symptoms varies, as does the frequency of the attacks of vertigo which may occur every few weeks or every few years. Some relief may be obtained from a variety of preparations but, in severe cases, it may be necessary to destroy part of the inner ear surgically.

Summary of nursing points

Epilepsy is a symptom of disease, and not a disease in itself. However, its high rate of occurrence (one person in two hundred is liable to be affected) means that the nurse will frequently be responsible for caring for a patient with this condition. The nurse's responsibility is to reassure the patient and, should an attack develop, prevent him from injuring himself. She must also observe him for loss of consciousness, convulsions, incontinence and the actual duration of the attack. She should note and report any observations made, as the information obtained may be important in helping the doctor to diagnose the cause of the condition and effect the correct treatment.

As always, the nurse must ensure that any treatment prescribed is carried out.

Chapter 9 Diseases of uncertain cause

Multiple (disseminated) sclerosis

This disorder is much more common in the temperate than in the tropical countries. The reason for this is uncertain, and its cause is unknown. In this condition there is a degeneration of the myelin sheath which surrounds the nerve axons in the brain and spinal cord – hence the name *demyelination*. The areas or *plaques* of demyelination may be single or multiple and they may occur in different parts of the central nervous system, either simultaneously or at different times. The neurological disturbance which follows is due to the fact that the axons which are involved in the demyelination fail to conduct nerve impulses, so that the patient develops paralysis or sensory or bladder disturbance, depending on which fibres are affected.

The characteristic features of the illness are attacks which last a few weeks and which are followed by complete or partial recovery of function. Characteristically, there are relapses and remissions. The word *disseminated* is used because the plaques are often disseminated in various parts of the central nervous system. The attacks are also disseminated in time, meaning that the patient usually suffers from recurrent episodes spread over many years. Most commonly an attack is characterized by the development of weakness, or pins-and-needles or numbness in one limb, or both lower limbs, or down one side of the body, depending on the exact situation of the plaque. Often, the plaque may involve the cerebellum or its connections with the brain-stem and then the patient has ataxia, dysarthria (slurred speech) and nystagmus (jerky eye movements). Double vision results from plaques of demyelination in the brain-stem.

Retrobulbar neuritis is the description given to the involvement of the optic nerve which produces loss of vision and discomfort in the eye on movement. (Disseminated sclerosis is a disease of the central nervous system and does not affect the peripheral nerves, but the optic nerve is really an extension of the brain and, in effect, is a part of the CNS.)

In most attacks the symptoms begin to disappear after six to eight weeks, but recovery may be only partial. There may never be recurrence, or there may be freedom from attacks for twenty or more years. Sometimes, however, the exacerbations may recur at an ever-increasing rate, with less and less recovery and time in between. Sometimes, too, the disease may progress without any remissions at all. There is no way of telling which patient is likely to belong to which of these groups. The unfortunate, with many attacks or no remissions, eventually become bedridden because of weakness or ataxia or both and easily develop pressure sores as a result of loss of sensation below the level of the plaque in the spinal cord. Bladder and rectal function are disturbed by the interruption of nerve fibres in the spinal cord. Patients may have frequency and urgency of micturition or develop a large painless bladder due to retention of urine, often followed by incontinence due to overflow.

Many theories have been proposed to account for the cause of this illness. In the past it has been attributed to poisoning by some unspecified toxic factor, infection by an unidentified microorganism and a variety of dietary deficiences. Currently, the possibility of infection with a slow virus is thought likely. This kind of virus is thought to lie dormant in nervous tissues and produce damage, either directly or through some kind of allergic or immune effect.

No cure for the condition exists, but the different symptoms may be relieved in a variety of ways. In acute attacks, corticosteroids may assist in speeding up recovery, and ACTH injections may be tried in short courses lasting three to four weeks. Long-term treatment with corticosteroids has not been found of value in preventing relapses. Weakness due to upper motor neurone lesions is usually accompanied by spasticity in the muscles involved. This may be relieved by a combination of physiotherapy and a variety of drugs, such as *diazepam* or *lioresal*. Severe spasticity of the muscles may result in deformities such as plantar flexion of the feet or drawing together of the thighs (*adduction*). In such severe cases, the tendons of the affected muscles may be cut (*tenotomy*) to relieve the spasm and thus make nursing the bedridden patient easier by enabling him to lie on his back (or front) and to sit in a chair, instead of being continuously confined to bed on his side. In order to achieve similar effect, the motor nerve roots to the spastic muscles of the legs may be destroyed by an injection of phenol through a lumbar-puncture needle (see Figure 41). Disturbance of bladder function is difficult to treat. Urgency and frequency due to spasm of bladder muscle may be relieved by certain smooth-muscle relaxants. There is unfortunately no cure for incontinence, other than the use of appropriate appliances in men. No effective appliance exists for women. In order to avoid persistent wetting, it may be preferable to use an indwelling catheter, though this is bound, after a time, to result in the introduction of infection into the bladder and ultimately the kidneys. This may be eradicated by the use of urinary antibiotics, but tends to recur.

When discussing disseminated sclerosis with patients and relations, it is important to remember and stress that the condition is very often mild and may be limited to only two or three attacks during a lifetime with good recovery from each. It is easy to overlook this when working in a hospital atmosphere and dealing only with the most severely affected patients with progressively increasing disabilities. The great majority of patients with this illness hardly ever require admission to hospital.

Cerebellar degeneration

A variety of disorders produce degeneration of the neurones and supporting cells in the cerebellum. They have slightly different features but the essential symptoms are ataxia, incoordination and dysarthria. Sometimes there is also nystagmus. Some of these disorders run in families and some may be associated with damage to the spinal cord or peripheral nerves. There is no specific treatment for any of them.

Motor neurone disease

This is a disease of unknown cause usually affecting men and women in the second half of life. The pathological lesion consists of degeneration of motor neurones in the cortex (upper motor neurones) and in the spinal cord (lower motor neurones), so that the patient presents with a mixed upper and lower motor neurone lesion. The former produces weakness, spasticity, increased tendon reflexes and an extensor plantar response whilst the latter produces muscle wasting and tends to diminish the tendon reflexes. When the condition affects the neurones in the brain-stem, bulbar palsy results, and there is *dysphagia* (difficulty in swallowing) and dysarthria. There is no known cure for this disorder, which tends to result in death within five to seven years of onset.

Dementia

Dementia usually occurs in the elderly, though occasionally it may be present in younger patients. Its main feature is intellectual deterioration, the chief symptom being impairment of memory. Other features may appear later; these include difficulty with speaking (dysphasia) and difficulty with performing such complex actions as getting dressed or striking a match even though there is no absence of normal power and coordination (a condition known as *apraxia*). The symptoms are due to a diffuse disorder affecting neurones throughout the cerebral cortex. In the elderly this may be due to arteriosclerosis causing death of neurones through chronic insufficiency of blood supply, or it may be a primary process known as *senile dementia*. In patients under the age of sixty-five, dementia is generally known as *presenile* and is usually due to a primary disorder of unknown cause called *Alzheimer's disease*.

It is important, whenever possible, to exclude treatable causes of dementia, such as neurosyphilis, vitamin B_{12} deficiency, myxoedema and certain brain tumours which may present as dementia, usually by producing chronic raised intracranial pressure. Unfortunately, once such conditions have been eliminated, nothing can be offered to the patient apart from sympathetic care.

Degenerative disorders of the spinal column

With increasing age, changes take place in the joints between vertebrae along the whole length of the spinal column. These joints between the vertebrae contain the intervertebral disc, which has a softish centre surrounded by cartilage and a fibrous capsule. Degenerative changes due

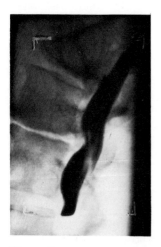

Figure 49 X-ray showing a lumbar disc protrusion outlined against myodil dye

to age, aggravated by trauma, result in the formation of excessive amounts of cartilage and this may protrude into the spinal canal and compress the spinal cord (Figure 49). It may also protrude laterally and press on nerve roots emerging from the spinal cord out of the spinal canal. This degenerative process is known as *spondylosis* and tends to occur particularly in the cervical and lumbar segments.

Cervical spondylosis (Figure 50) may produce local neck pain, root symptoms in the arms consisting of pain, weakness, numbness and pins-and-needles (*paraesthesiae*), or symptoms of spinal cord compression affecting the legs and bladder. *Lumbar spondylosis* may produce back pain (*lumbago*). By compressing the roots of the sciatic nerve, spondylosis may also cause severe pain down the back of the leg (*sciatica*).

Treatment
This depends on which particular symptoms are most troublesome. Local and root pain respond to rest, because this reduces movement at the joints. The neck or lumbar spine may be immobilized in the appropriate collar or belt, and rest in bed may be essential.

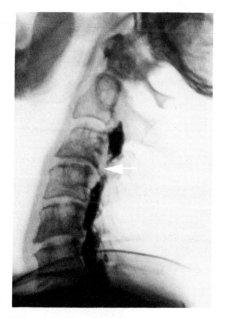

Figure 50 X-ray showing cervical spondylosis; the filling defect is arrowed

More persistent or severe lesions may require surgical treatment. In the cervical region this consists of the removal of the posterior part of the vertebral body (the *lamina*) to give the spinal cord more room and perhaps the fusion (joining) of two or more vertebrae to stabilize them by means of a bone graft. In the lumbar region, it may be possible to remove the prolapsed part of the intervertebral disc which has produced root compression. There is no doubt that sometimes low back pain is relieved by a variety of manipulative procedures, but these are positively dangerous if carried out on the cervical spine and may result in complete paralysis of all four limbs (*quadriplegia*) because of damage to the cervical spinal cord.

Syringomyelia

This is a rare disorder of the spinal cord in which, for reasons not clearly understood, a cavity forms within the centre of the cord usually in the cervical area. This results in the interruption of the sensory fibres concerned with the sensation of pain and temperature (Figure 51). At the level where they enter through the sensory root, these fibres cross to the opposite side of the spinal cord before ascending to the cerebral hemisphere. Loss of pain and temperature sensation with preservation of touch sensation in the area of the skin affected (because the 'touch' sensory fibres ascend the cord without crossing over) is known as *dissociated sensory loss*. In such patients, it is usual for the hands to be first affected and painless burns and ulcers develop on the fingers, which may become gangrenous and require amputation.

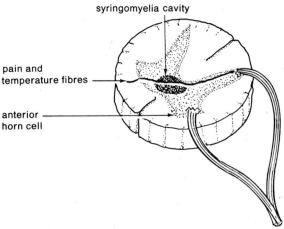

Figure 51 Syringomyelia

The cavity in the cord also affects the anterior horn cells at that level, producing wasting and weakness of the muscles supplied by these neurones. Eventually the cavity expands to destroy the descending upper motor neurone and ascending sensory fibres, producing weakness and sensory loss below. There is no specific treatment for this disease, but surgical measures can help by decompressing the cord and draining the fluid-filled cavity.

Parkinsonism

This term describes a disorder which affects the basal ganglia, a collection of neurones lying deep in the cerebral hemispheres. It produces three main symptoms: tremor, rigidity and *akinesia*. Akinesia, a very disabling symptom, describes poverty of movement, and inability to perform actions. This feature is not directly due to the tremor or the rigidity, nor to any weakness.

The cause of the great majority of cases of parkinsonism is unknown. However, some patients develop the condition as a result of an attack of encephalitis, and this was a very important cause after a world-wide epidemic of *encephalitis lethargica*, which occurred around 1920. Parkinsonism may also sometimes occur as a toxic side-effect caused by certain drugs of the *phenothiazine* variety (such as chlorpromazine) and by *reserpine*, a drug once much used for the treatment of high blood pressure.

A condition like parkinsonism may occur in patients with cerebrovascular disease who have had multiple small infarcts in the region of the basal ganglia and brain-stem. These patients present with a mixture of upper motor neurone (or *pyramidal*) and basal ganglia (or *extra-pyramidal*) features.

Parkinson's disease (or *idiopathic parkinsonism*) is the most common cause of the disorder. It affects men and women, usually beginning in the sixth decade. The tremor, which affects particularly the fingers and hands, is sometimes described as 'pill rolling'. The akinesia is responsible for the poverty of facial expression and of movements such as blinking – hence the typical 'mask-like' face. Patients have difficulty with initiating movements such as walking and fail to swing their arms when they do so. Once walking, they may have difficulty in stopping, and tend to shuffle along with rapid little steps: the voice becomes weak and monotonous and handwriting becomes smaller and generally deteriorates.

Treatment

The medical treatment of parkinsonism is based on the observation that the disabilities are due to an imbalance between the chemical actions of substances transmitting messages between neurones, for instance *acetylcholine*, which is overactive, and *dopamine*, of which there is a deficiency. This can be counteracted by administering drugs which diminish the action of acetylcholine or those which increase the amount of dopamine in the central nervous system. An example of the former is *benzhexol* (Artane), which can be given by mouth. Like other drugs of this group, benzhexol may produce dryness of the mouth and occasionally drowsiness and confusion. Dopamine can be increased in the basal ganglia by giving *L-Dopa* by mouth. This may produce nausea, anorexia and hypotension with giddiness and it is usual to give a small dose initially and increase it every few days until the drug produces the maximum benefit, or until side-effects occur. Occasionally, long-continued administration of L-Dopa may itself produce involuntary movement and the dose may then have to be reduced or the drug stopped altogether.

Surgical lesions in the basal ganglia have been found to relieve the symptoms of parkinsonism on the side opposite to the operation. The procedure is carried out by the so-called *stereotactic technique*. The position of the basal ganglia is calculated from models of the skull and the brain; through small holes in the skull bones, wires are inserted so that areas around the basal ganglia can be coagulated electrically. This method produces good results, though there is always a risk of affecting the speech or producing hemiplegia, since other areas of the brain could be damaged inadvertently. Since the discovery of L-Dopa, the stereotactic operation has been used much less.

Patients with parkinsonism benefit from physiotherapy. They are also helped by such simple measures as wearing slip-on shoes instead of lace-up shoes and using zip-fasteners instead of buttons wherever possible.

Other disorders of the basal ganglia

Extra-apyramidal disorders result in a variety of involuntary movements. *Chorea* is characterized by jerky purposeless movements which may involve the limbs, body or face. It occurs in several diseases. *Rheumatic* or *Sydenham's* chorea is a childhood disorder which is believed to be related to rheumatic fever. Occasionally a similar condition occurs during pregnancy and is known as *chorea gravidarum*. It has also been described in women on the contraceptive pill. *Huntington's chorea* is a totally different hereditary disorder which presents late in life in association with progressive dementia. *Athetosis* is a writhing snake-like movement involving the limbs and occasionally the trunk and facial muscles. It may occur in association with chorea, in children with brain damage sustained during intra-uterine life or at birth, when it is then known as *choreo-athetosis*.

Summary of nursing points

The condition of multiple sclerosis has been given much prominence in recent years; this is due to its relatively high rate of incidence and to its debilitating and demoralizing effects on a person. The nursing care and management of the patient, particularly during the advanced stages of the disease, calls for dedication and a high degree of nursing skills. Important points in the nursing management include improving morale and preventing skin lesions, such as pressure sores. The patient should be nursed on a ripple bed during the acute stage of the illness, and all methods that are feasible must be used to prevent pressure sores. The patient should be turned regularly, the skin kept dry and a barrier cream applied. If the patient is incontinent of urine, then catheterization or tidal drainage may be indicated. An adequate diet must be given which is rich in vitamins, roughage-containing foods, fluid and sufficient protein.

The nurse, by her attitude and relationship with the patient, should do everything possible to make him feel secure and happy.

Further reading

General
Books

E. R. Bickerstaff, *Neurology for Nurses*, 2nd edn, English Universities Press, 1971. A comprehensive account of the nervous system. Includes clinical signs of disorder, and treatment of individual diseases.

W. R. Brain, *Clinical Neurology*, 4th edn, revised by R. Bannister, Oxford University Press, 1973. A book for reference, giving an account of signs and symptoms of neurological disorders, detailed descriptions of diseases and treatment.

J. Marshall, and Jean Mair, *Neurological Nursing : A Practical Guide*, Blackwell Scientific, 1967. Not an account of diseases, but a detailed description of the care of a patient with neurological disorder.

W. B. Matthews, and H. Miller, *Diseases of the Nervous System*, Blackwell, 1972. A detailed but clear account of the diseases – primarily for doctors, but good for reference for nurses.

Chapter 1 The structure and function of the nervous system
Books

E. R. Bickerstaff, *Neurology for Nurses*, 2nd edn, English Universities Press, 1971. Chapter 3 gives a clear and concise account of the structure and function of the nervous system.

W. R. Brain, *Clinical Neurology*, 4th edn, revised by R. Bannister, Oxford University Press, 1973. The introduction outlines the approach to neurological diagnosis, and gives a statement of the steps in neurological examination.

J. Gibson, *A Guide to the Nervous System*, 2nd edn, Faber, 1967. An illustrated account of the structure and function of the nervous system – an introduction to the subject.

W. Hewitt, *Functional Neuroanatomy*, *Nursing Times*, 1972. A simple and clear account of the structure of the nervous system and its function, with many helpful illustrations.

A. E. Hugh, *Nervous System and Endocrine Glands*, Butterworth, 1971. A presentation of facts with revision summary paragraphs as learning exercises.

J. N. Walton, *Essentials of Neurology*, 3rd edn, Pitman Medical, 1971. Chapter 1 gives some general principles in neurology with the main groups of disorders and the foundations of their recognition.

Chapter 2 The pathology of neurological disorders
Books

E. R. Bickerstaff, *Neurology for Nurses*, 2nd edn, English Universities Press, 1971. Chapter 4 describes clinical signs of damage to nervous tissue, while chapter 18 outlines what the nurse needs to know about investigation of the nervous system.

G. Holmes, *Introduction to Clinical Neurology*, 3rd edn, revised by W. B. Matthews, Churchill Livingstone, 1968. Chapters 1 to 3 give a clear but concise account of the signs and symptoms of neurological disorder, with the underlying pathology, and the methods adopted in examining the patient.

U. Jolly, *Lumbar Puncture and Related Tests*, Butterworth, 1972. The basic knowledge needed for a nurse to understand lumbar puncture and other related tests, and her role in the procedure.

J. N. Walton, *Essentials of Neurology*, 3rd edn, Pitman Medical, 1971. Chapters 1 to 3 give a detailed account of neurological disorders and the investigations carried out to establish diagnosis.

Articles

P. M. Davies, 'Practical neurological assessment', *Physiotherapy*, vol. 58, Dec. 1972, pp. 106–109. A suggested method of carrying out this assessment – compiled for physiotherapists treating patients with neurological disorders.

P. M. Jeavons, 'Electroencephalography', *Nursing Times*, vol. 67, 28 Jan. 1971, pp. 106–109. An explanation of how electroencephalography works and how the nurse, by preparing the patient, can help the technician get a good recording.

Chapter 3 Cerebrovascular disorders
Books

W. R. Brain, *Clinical Neurology*, 4th edn, revised by R. Bannister, Oxford University Press, 1973. Chapter 8 briefly describes temporal arteritis, its origin, symptoms and treatment.

A. B. Carter, *All About Strokes*, Nelson, 1968. An account of what happens in a stroke, how it may be caused, prevented, and how treated. A lot of facts in an easily digested form.

V. E. Griffith, *A Stroke in the Family*, Penguin, 1970. How a patient can be brought back to useful and enjoyable life after a stroke. Some useful methods and advice.

P. E. Jay, E. Walker and A. Ellison, *Help Yourselves: a Handbook for Hemiplegics and Their Families*, 2nd edn, Butterworth, 1972. How to do all the ordinary and necessary things of life. Really practical instruction.

W. B. Jennett, *An Introduction to Neurosurgery*, 2nd edn, Heinemann, 1970. Chapter 16 is useful as reference material for nurses, though the book is written for doctors. Gives pathology, symptoms and outline of treatment.

J. Marshall, *The Management of Cerebrovascular Disease*, Churchill, 1965. Though written for doctors, this book provides useful material for reference. It gives principles governing new approaches to strokes – their diagnosis and management.

D. Ritchie, *Stroke: A Diary of Recovery*, Faber, 1960. A patient describing, quite subjectively, his return to health after a stroke, with all the care, treatment and help he received.

T. Wareham, *Return to Independence: Exercises for Stroke Patients*, 2nd edn, Chest and Heart Association, 1970. A booklet for the help and guidance of those who suffer a stroke, and for anyone concerned with their recovery.

Articles

G. F. Adams, 'Principles of the treatment of stroke', *Nursing Mirror*, vol. 135, 7 July 1972, pp. 12–13. A clear and sympathetic account of the treatment of a patient suffering a stroke, with consideration of the specific handicaps which may delay recovery and the basic principles underlying treatment.

M. E. Alcock, 'Recovery from "stroke"', *District Nursing*, vol. 3, May 1972, pp. 30–31. An account of a patient's recovery at home.

J. Bowers, 'Counter-stroke: Patient's experiences of rehabilitation after a stroke', *Occupational Therapy*, vol. 35, May 1972, pp. 315–17. The author emphasizes in this simple record of her experience how much occupational therapy helped in her rehabilitation.

J. C. Brocklehurst, 'Guidelines for rehabilitating stroke patients 1: Dysphasia and the nurse', *Nursing Mirror*, vol. 133, 22 Oct. 1971, pp. 17–19. The processes involved in speech and speech disorders, and the function of the speech therapist.

A. W. Brompton, 'Stroke rehabilitation', *Nursing Times*, vol. 59, 5 July 1963, pp. 828–30. A district nurse describes how a patient, with the help of his family and the home nursing service, can return to independence at home.

A. E. Holmes, 'Cerebral aneurysm', *Nursing Times*, vol. 68, 22 June 1972, pp. 777–80. An account of the nature of aneurysms, their dangers and symptoms, with treatment and management.

L. J. Hurwitz, 'Management of major strokes', *British Medical Journal*, vol. 3, 20 Sept. 1969, pp. 699–701. A clear account of the management, treatment and aftercare of patients suffering from a stroke.

E. C. Hutchinson, 'Little strokes', *British Medical Journal*, vol. 4, 4 Oct. 1969, pp. 32–5. Brief vascular attacks – their causes and management, including hypoglycaemia.

P. M. Kimber, and G. A. Morgan, 'Cerebral angiography by arterial catheterization', *Nursing Times*, vol. 66, 3 Sept. 1970, pp. 1137–40. The use of this technique in investigating cerebrovascular disease, the method used and the care of the patient both before and after this procedure.

D. P. Leisten, 'Rehabilitation of hemiplegics in the home', *Nursing Times*, vol. 61, 23 July 1965, pp. 1004–1006. An account of the way a district nurse can continue the rehabilitation of a patient at home after discharge from hospital, with programme and illustrations.

S. P. Meadows, 'Subarachnoid haemorrhage', *Nursing Mirror*, vol. 132, 4 June 1971, pp. 19–23. A detailed account of the condition and other types of intracranial haemorrhage, its clinical features, investigations and care of the patient.

J. Mitchell, 'Guidelines for rehabilitating stroke patients 2: Early management of the aphasic patient', *Nursing Mirror*, vol. 133, 22 Oct. 1971, pp. 19–21. The practical help that can be given by the nurse.

I. F. Pye, 'Lesions in cerebrovascular disease', *Nursing Mirror*, vol. 135, 11 Aug. 1972, pp. 15–16. The present-day approach to the miscellaneous conditions responsible for the stroke syndrome.

S. Rubin, 'Home care of the stroke patient', *Nursing Times*, vol. 63, 6 Oct. 1967, pp. 1339, 1342–3. An account of the way in which a patient can not only learn and be helped to cope with his disability at home, but can even improve his condition.

Chapter 4 Tumours of the nervous system
Books

E. R. Bickerstaff, *Neurology for Nurses*, 2nd edn, English Universities Press, 1971. Chapter 8 gives general features of cerebral tumours; the direct effect of raised pressure on the brain; different kinds of tumours and how diagnosis is arrived at. Brief account of spinal tumours and tumours of peripheral nerves.

W. R. Brain, *Clinical Neurology*, 4th edn, revised by R. Bannister, Oxford University Press, 1973. Chapter 9 describes intracranial tumours – how tumours arise, their mode of onset, and the symptoms they may cause, the investigations which are carried out, prognosis, and outline of treatment.

W. B. Jennett, *An Introduction to Neurosurgery*, 2nd edn, Heinemann, 1970. Chapter 1 and chapters 4 to 9 are useful for reference; they give details of signs and symptoms, clinical diagnosis, investigation and treatment of brain tumours. Chapter 15 describes spinal tumours, investigation, effects and treatment.

W. B. Matthews, and H. Miller, *Diseases of the Nervous System*, Blackwell, 1972. Chapter 8 gives a clear account of the effects and causes of raised intracranial pressure, the clinical features, diagnosis and treatment of cerebral tumours. Chapter 9 describes tumours of the spinal cord.

Articles

E. R. Bickerstaff, 'Brain-stem tumours', *Nursing Times*, vol. 65, 20 Nov. 1969, pp. 1488–91. The clinical features, investigation and treatment of tumours of this vital part of the brain. Prognosis and some thoughts on management and prolongation of life.

J. E. Fretwell, 'Nursing care study. A child dies', *Nursing Times*, vol. 69, 5 July 1973, pp. 867–71. Detailed account describing the signs and symptoms and the whole course of the illness (a case of glioma of the thalamus), with treatment.

R. A. Henson, 'Neurological manifestations of malignant disease', *Nursing Mirror*, vol. 129, 26 Sept. 1969, pp. 29–31. A consideration of the effects on the nervous system of malignant disease elsewhere in the body.

Chapter 5 Head injuries
Books

R. Hooper, *Patterns of Acute Head Injury*, Edward Arnold, 1969. Designed for reading basic principles from which management can be evolved, this book is written for doctors but provides a reference book for nurses.

K. G. Jamieson, *A First Notebook of Head Injury*, 2nd edn, Butterworth, 1971. A concise yet detailed account of injuries which may be sustained, their clinical course, and the care and management of the patient.

W. Lewin, *The Management of Head Injuries*, Baillière, Tindall & Cassell, 1966. Written for doctors but a useful reference book, giving comprehensive information on practical aspects of care specific to patients with head injuries.

P. S. London (ed.), *Modern Trends in Accident Surgery and Medicine*, Butterworth, 1970. Chapter 6 gives some of the medical, social and personal problems of those surviving severe head injury – with case histories.

P. S. London, *Nursing Emergencies*, Blackwell, 1967. Chapter 5 gives an account of the surgical treatment of head injuries with the nursing care and management of the unconscious patient.

T. S. Mann, W. H. Reid, A. B. N. Telfer and R. Tyn, *Accident Surgery for Nurses*, Livingstone, 1969. Chapter 6 gives an explanation of the principles on which management is based, with suggestions for special nursing care and observation.

L. W. Plewes (ed.), *Accident Service*, Pitman, 1966. Chapter 4 describes the recognition and emergency treatment of head injuries. Although written for doctors, the part on management (pp. 69–71) is especially useful for the nurse.

J. M. Potter, *The Practical Management of Head Injuries*, Lloyd-Luke, 1961. A practical guide to the care of patients with head injuries – in the casualty department and ward. Written for the doctor, but of use for reference to the nurse.

H. Proctor and P. S. London, *Principles of First Aid for the Injured*, 2nd edn, Butterworth, 1968. Intended for doctors, chapter 9 describes the different injuries and their results, and indicates important aspects of treatment from the first-aid point of view.

P. A. Ring, *The Care of the Injured*, 2nd edn, Churchill Livingstone, 1969. Chapter 4 gives a brief but clear account of head injuries, their management and care.

Articles

A. G. Austin, 'Social work with head injury patients', *Medical Social Work*, vol. 22, Feb. 1970, pp. 310–18. An account of the work of the Birmingham Accident Hospital staff with head-injury patients, showing the sphere of social work in helping with their problems.

F. E. Bruckner, and A. P. H. Randle, 'Return to work after severe head injuries', *Rheumatology and Physical Medicine*, vol. 11, Aug. 1972, pp. 344–8. A discussion of the patient's problems and those of his family and society, with a plan for rehabilitation.

P. N. Knight, 'Rehabilitation of head injuries', *Nursing Mirror*, vol. 136, 30 March 1973, pp. 14–19. Various forms of treatment used in the rehabilitation of patients after severe head injury, with measures and equipment used to help them regain independence.

H. Proctor, 'Head injuries and the problems faced by the crippled survivors', *Physiotherapy*, vol. 55, Mar. 1969, pp. 93–7. Some of the problems and disabilities faced by patients after head injuries, with treatment and resettlement.

Chapter 6 Infections of the nervous system
Books

E. R. Bickerstaff, *Neurology for Nurses*, 2nd edn, English Universities Press, 1971. Chapter 7 describes infection and inflammation of the nervous system, and gives a concise classification of the forms of infection, with general features, symptoms and in some cases (e.g. poliomyelitis) treatment and prevention.

W. R. Brain, *Clinical Neurology*, 4th edn, revised by R. Bannister, Oxford University Press, 1973. Part 3, chapters 20 to 23, gives a detailed account of infection in the nervous system – scholarly but clear. Deals with encephalitis, poliomyelitis, meningitis and syphilis.

R. D. Catterall, *Venereology for Nurses: A Textbook of the Sexually Transmitted Diseases*, English Universities Press, 1964. Chapter 5 gives facts about neurosyphilis, its manifestations, symptoms, investigation and prognosis.

H. Elliott, and K. Ryz, *Venereal Diseases: Treatment and Nursing*, Baillière Tindall, 1972. Chapter 4 gives a short account of neurosyphilis, the signs and symptoms, prognosis and treatment.

A. King, and C. Nicol, *Venereal Diseases*, 2nd edn, Baillière, Tindall & Cassell, 1969. Chapter 5 gives a detailed account of neurosyphilis, different types, their diagnosis, treatment and sequelous involvement of meninges and blood vessels.

J. N. Walton, *Essentials of Neurology*, 3rd edn, Pitman Medical, 1971. Chapter 14 gives a detailed account of infection and the nervous system, including neurological complications of specific infections. Suitable for senior nurses.

Articles

L. Bokhoree, 'Nursing care study. Chronic otogenic cerebral abscess', *Nursing Times*, vol. 69, 22 Feb. 1973, pp. 236–7. An account of the illness of a patient whose headache was found to be due to a large cerebral abscess, and treated by craniotomy, drainage and antibiotics, until fit to be discharged home.

T. H. Flewett, 'Acute polyneuritis', *Nursing Times*, vol. 68, 2 March 1972, pp. 266–7. An account of the condition and its complications. Comparison with poliomyelitis and other forms of polyneuritis. Some points of nursing care.

G. Malembeka, 'Nursing care study. Meningitis', *Nursing Times*, vol. 69, 22 Feb. 1973, pp. 241–2. Description of the illness and treatment of a child in Tanzania. No facilities for culture were available and several false diagnoses were made. Once that of meningitis had been made and treatment for this started, the baby began to improve and recovered.

W. Sharp, *et al.*, 'Control of an outbreak of meningococcal meningitis in a day school', *Community Medicine*, vol. 129, 15 Dec. 1972, pp. 211–12. An account of the measures taken including post-nasal swabbing of contacts, chemoprophylaxis with assessment of antibody levels; full cooperation of staff, pupils and parents.

L. Stewart, 'Meningitis at age 4 weeks', *Nursing Mirror*, vol. 135, 7 July 1972, pp. 30–32. A nursing care study of a baby with severe meningitis who made a good recovery. A brief summary of the common varieties of meningitis.

Chapter 7 Disorders of peripheral nerves and muscles
Articles

M. E. Biley, 'Nursing care study. Transient myasthenia gravis in the new born', *Nursing Mirror*, vol. 136, 30 March 1973, pp. 24–6. A description of the cause of the condition and the detailed care of a newborn baby.

J. M. Courtney, 'Patient care study: myasthenia gravis', *Queen's Nursing Journal*, vol. 16, April 1973, pp. 11–12. An account of a patient with this disease, her care at home, and thoughts on the disorder from the patient's point of view.

A. E. E. Emery, 'Muscular dystrophies', *Nursing Mirror*, vol. 126, 1 March 1968, pp. 26–8. An account of the different types of muscular dystrophy.

T. H. Flewett, 'Acute polyneuritis', *Nursing Times*, vol. 68, 2 March 1972, pp. 266–7. An account of the different kinds of polyneuritis, their causes, complications and nursing care.

P. A. Turner, 'Case study. Muscular dystrophy (the role of the district nurse)', *District Nursing*, vol. 15, 7 Oct. 1972, pp. 147–9. Care of a patient in the home.

J. M. Walton, 'Muscular dystrophies and their management', *British Medical Journal*, vol. 3, 13 Sept. 1969, pp. 639–42. A classification of muscular dystrophies, their diagnosis, treatment and management with special reference to genetic considerations.

Chapter 8 Paroxysmal disorders
Books

Central Health Services Council, *People with Epilepsy*, Report of a joint sub-committee of the Standing Medical Advisory Committee and Advisory Committee on the Health and Welfare of Handicapped Persons, HMSO, 1969. A review of the scope of available services for epileptic people and some suggestions for future development.

Friedreich's Ataxia Group, *Friedreich's Ataxia : A Handbook for Patients and Relatives*, Friedreich's Ataxia Group, 1972. Simple practical advice for patients with addresses for getting special help and advice.

K. M. Hay, *Do Something About That Migraine*, Tandem, 1968. Some information (for sufferers) on the nature of migraine, what may cause it and how it can be relieved.

Migraine Trust, *Focus on Migraine*, Migraine Trust, 1971. A pamphlet giving a concise account of what migraine is, what brings it on, warning signs and medical treatment.

Articles

M. Barrie, 'Migraine – a disabling disorder', *Nursing Times*, vol. 68, May 1972, pp. 640–42. A simple account of the disease and its treatment and prevention.

M. Bartha, 'Chalfont centre for epilepsy', *Nursing Times*, vol. 69, 15 March 1973, pp. 332–5. The work of a centre for the care and rehabilitation of patients with epilepsy.

K. S. W. Brennan, 'Epilepsy', *Nursing Times*, vol. 67, 15 April 1971, pp. 435–8. The investigation and treatment of epilepsy and the problems of its sufferers in society.

G. S. Burden, 'Social aspects of epilepsy', *Occupational Health*, vol. 17, July/Aug. 1965, pp. 205–209. Employment difficulties of epileptics. Facts about accident liability.

J. D. Carroll, 'Migraine – general management', *British Medical Journal*, 1971, vol. 2, 8 Oct. 1971, pp. 756–7. Factors which aggravate migraine – ways to prevent attacks.

J. B. Cook, 'Status epilepticus', *Nursing Mirror*, vol. 126, 22 March 1967, pp. 18–19. An account of the condition, its treatment and nursing care.

W. Dawson, 'The British Epilepsy Association and what it is doing for epileptics and their families', *Nursing Times*, vol. 67, 15 April 1971, p. 440. The needs of epileptics and how the Society likes to meet them.

D. Denham, 'Nursing care study. Endolymphatic shunt for the treatment of Ménière's disease', *Nursing Times*, vol. 68, 12 Oct. 1972, pp. 1287–8. An account of a patient having surgical treatment for Ménière's disease, with details of the operation.

District Nursing, 'Finding jobs for epileptics', *District Nursing*, vol. 11, Aug. 1968, pp. 99–101. The possibility of employment under normal conditions for epileptics. Some unsuitable kinds of work, and many suitable kinds.

J. B. Foster, 'Facial pain', *Nursing Mirror*, vol. 135, 28 July 1972, pp. 25–7. A classification of neurogenic facial pain including post-herpetic neuralgia, trigeminal neuralgia and migrainous neuralgia, etc.

J. A. Furness, 'Methods of treating acute migraine in the City Migraine Clinic', *Nursing Times*, vol. 67, 8 April 1971, pp. 414–15. A report of the first year's work at the Clinic with a summary of the treatment given.

F. B. Gibberd, 'Epilepsy', *British Medical Journal*, vol. 4, 1 Nov. 1969, pp. 281–2. The management of epilepsy – control of fits and the social care of the patient.

J. Goodall, 'Convulsions in babies and young children', *Nursing Times*, vol. 65, 18 Sept. 1969, pp. 1195–6. All the conditions which may produce convulsions in babies. Dealing with the family.

T. K. Hardy, 'Post-herpetic neuralgia', *Nursing Mirror*, vol. 136, 22 June 1973, pp. 30–31. An account of the nature of the condition, a description of the type of pain, and some forms of treatment.

P. M. Jeavons, 'Television epilepsy', *Nursing Mirror*, vol. 135, 18 Aug. 1972, pp. 24–5. The effect of flickering lights on epileptics.

Lancet, 'Coping with epilepsy', *Lancet*, vol. 2, 12 Aug. 1972, p. 316. The case for social centres with social workers as well as medical personnel to help patients.

J. Manuel, 'Epilepsy in industry', *Occupational Health*, vol. 23, no. 3, March 1971, pp. 93–5. Problems of employment and the need for education of management and trade unions. The role of the nurse in this.

N. Mayne, 'Migraine', *Nursing Times*, vol. 64, 27 Sept. 1968, pp. 1294–5. An account of migraine, the onset of the attack, treatment and investigations.

M. Parsonage, 'Modern treatment of epilepsy', *Occupational Health*, vol. 17, July/Aug. 1965, pp. 202–205. The modern attitude to epilepsy, its investigation, medical and surgical treatment.

M. Parsonage, 'Modern management of epilepsy', *Nursing Mirror*, vol. 130, 3 Oct. 1969, pp. 34–8. An account of the nature and causation of epilepsy, types of seizure, treatment and general management.

M. Parsonage, 'Treatment of management of epilepsy', *District Nursing*, vol. 11, Aug. 1968, pp. 94–5. Clinical appraisal and investigation of epileptics, their medical and surgical treatment and management.

J. A. Simpson, 'Epilepsy', *Nursing Mirror*, vol. 137, 6 July 1972, pp. 27–9. An account of the nature of the disease, types of seizures, their observation and treatment.

R. Udall, 'Be grateful you're epileptic', *Nursing Times*, vol. 67, 15 April 1971. An account by a young epileptic of her life, illness and problems, and how she dealt with them.

M. C. Wall, 'Ergotamine tartrate in migraine and the dangers of overdose', *Nursing Times*, vol. 68, 14 Dec. 1972, p. 1585. A discussion of the findings of a study of patients with signs of overdose of the drug.

M. Wilkinson, 'Migraine – treatment of acute attack', *British Medical Journal*, vol. 2, 26 June 1971, pp. 754–5. A summary of drugs used to treat attacks and their methods of administration.

Chapter 9 Diseases of uncertain cause
Books

R. B. Godwin-Austen, *Parkinson's Disease : A Booklet for Patients and Their Families*, Parkinson's Disease Society, 1972. Concise account of what it is, what causes it, progress of the disease and how it is treated today.

Multiple Sclerosis Society, *At Home with Multiple Sclerosis*, Multiple Sclerosis Society, 1970. A summary of talks given to relatives of patients on different aspects of care and management.

Multiple Sclerosis Society, *Still at Home with Multiple Sclerosis*, Multiple Sclerosis Society, 1972. A further selection of talks to relatives, with information and advice.

Office of Health Economics, *Epilepsy in Society*, Office of Health Economics, 1971. Some interesting facts and statistics.

Office of Health Economics, *Migraine*, Office of Health Economics, 1972. History, prevalence and incidence of migraine concisely given, with characteristics of sufferers and the treatment of the disease.

L. Oliver, *Parkinson's Disease*, Heinemann, 1967. A detailed account of the condition, intended for doctors but valuable for reference. Gives the scientific basis of the syndrome, medical and surgical treatment.

G. Onuaguluchi, *Parkinsonism*, Butterworth, 1964. A detailed and scientific account of the disease – gives a clear and simple description of causes and factors influencing its development.

Articles

B. Ashworth, 'Multiple sclerosis', *District Nursing*, vol. 13, Feb. 1971, pp. 216–19. Modern ideas on the cause of this disease. Treatment and prevention of relapses and management of disability.

Assistant Hospital Secretary, 'Motor-neurone disease', *Nursing Times*, vol. 65, March 1969, pp. 300–304. An account by a patient of the problems and difficulties of sufferers of this disease and the ways in which a nurse can ease the lot of the patient.

D. B. Calne, 'L-Dopa and Parkinsonism', *Nursing Mirror*, vol. 133, 8 Oct. 1971, pp. 26–7. A brief account of the history of L-Dopa in the treatment of Parkinsonism.

D. Colver, 'Multiple sclerosis', *Nursing Times*, vol. 69, 3 May 1973, pp. 565–7. The story of this patient's struggle to live normally with her disease. This is followed by an account of the disease, its clinical features, prognosis and treatment – with the help of Social Services.

P. Cooper, 'Advances in the treatment of Parkinsonism', *Midwife and Health Visitor*, vol. 8, June 1972, p. 220. A clear account of the recent changes and treatment and the use of modern drugs.

R. H. Johnson, and D. L. McLellan, 'Multiple sclerosis', *Practitioner*, vol. 209, Aug. 1972, pp. 183–90. A short account of aetiology, early clinical features, prognosis, aids to diagnosis, treatment and community services – meant for doctors but useful for nurses.

J. B. Lyon, 'A case of multiple sclerosis', *Nursing Times*, vol. 67, 23 Dec. 1971, pp. 1601–602. The pathology, clinical picture, causes and treatment of the disease, with information about the first case ever recorded.

D. McAlpine, 'Multiple sclerosis: a review', *British Medical Journal*, vol. 2, 5 May 1973, pp. 292–5. Recent progress in knowledge of the disease, recognition and medico-social care. Comprehensive but clearly described.

J. H. D. Millar, 'Multiple sclerosis', *Nursing Times*, vol. 63, 27 Oct. 1967, pp. 1438–9. A short account of the disease, treatment, nursing care and social care.

Occupational Therapy, an issue entirely devoted to Parkinson's disease, vol. 35, Nov. 1972. A series of papers by specialists on subjects including diagnosis, medical aspects and treatment, surgical treatment, functional assessment, and how to live with the condition.

C. A. Pallis, 'Parkinsonism: natural history and clinical features', *British Medical Journal*, vol. 3, 18 Sept. 1971, pp. 683–90. A detailed account of the disease, its history, clinical features and diagnosis.

J. D. Parkes, 'Parkinson's disease', *District Nursing*, vol. 13, Feb. 1971, pp. 214–15. The history and nature of the disease, and new hope for treatment with modern drugs.

M. Redden, 'Paralysis agitans and L-Dopa drug therapy', *Nursing Times*, vol. 68, 2 March 1972, pp. 262–5. A nursing care study of a patient treated with L-Dopa. The patient is described in detail, his illness and treatment.

W. R. Russell, 'Multiple sclerosis', *Nursing Mirror*, vol. 135, 29 Dec. 1972, pp. 24–5. A description of some possible causes and mechanisms of multiple sclerosis, and some advice to sufferers.

G. Stern, 'Parkinsonism', *British Medical Journal*, vol. 4, 29 Nov. 1969, pp. 541–2. Recognition of the condition in its early stages. Modern forms of treatment by drugs and surgery.

B. Thompson, 'Parkinson people and others. Basic nursing of patients with mid-brain damage', *Nursing Times*, vol. 66, 6 Aug. 1970, pp. 1004–1006. An experienced nurse's understanding of the problems of these patients shows in this account of their care and management.

Acknowledgements

We wish to thank the following for permission to use material that has been the basis for some of the illustrations.

For Figure 6, 13, 25, 28, 31, 33, 39 and 40: English Universities Press Ltd, *Neurology for Nurses* (2nd edn) by Edwin R. Bickerstaff. For Figure 24 and 42: Orbis Publishing Company, *Mind and Body*. For Figure 43: Baillière Tindall, *Anatomy and Physiology for Nurses* (8th edn) by K. F. Armstrong and S. M. Jackson. For Figure 36: Dr J. Patten, *Neurology in Pictures* by Dr J. Patten. For Figure 41: Dr J. Patten, *Teach-In*.

Figures 17 and 48: photographs by Peter G. Tucker.

Index